My Operation

A Health Insider Becomes a P

My Operation

A Health Insider Becomes a Patient

Sholom Glouberman

Health and Everything Publications
Toronto, Ontario

© Health and Everything Publications 2010
Toronto, Ontario

Printed in the United States

ISBN 978-0-9812618-0-5 (paperback)

Library and Archives Canada Cataloguing in Publication

Glouberman, S.
My operation: a health insider becomes a patient /
Sholom Glouberman.

ISBN 978-0-9812618-0-5

1. Glouberman, S--Health. 2. Colectomy. 3. Operations,
Surgical. 4. Hospital care--Ontario--Toronto. 5. Hospital
patients--Ontario--Toronto. I. Title.

RD543.C57G56 2010   617.5'547092   C2010-902358-7

For Susan, with me always.

Contents

Foreword

This book is about a dilemma. By just about all counts, we are healthier than we have ever been before, no matter how we define "we," whether as mankind as a whole or particular segments thereof, divided as the developed or undeveloped world, as the wealthy or poor, by nationality or race. All generally accepted health care indices – life expectancy, infant mortality, whatever we can count – have improved over the years and seem to be still improving.

Our health care technology seems to know no bounds. We have antibiotics to control most acute infections and mini-invasive, even robotic surgery to patch up the wear and tear on vital organs. We can peer into every orifice and cranny of the body and discover all sorts of new diseases (hypertension, hypercholesterolemia, attention deficit disorder) that we never even knew we had before. What we can't cure (like diabetes or acquired immunodeficiency syndrome) we can keep under control with modern maintenance therapy.

We should rejoice in this progress, but somehow we don't seem to be as happy with our health care as we would like to be – as the evidence says that we should be. We have the uncomfortable feeling that just as many people die as ever before, only it takes longer and costs more. We sense that our health care system is in hot water and that maybe it is getting hotter. And maybe we're right.

A long time ago, but still well within historical time, our concepts of health and health care were more solidly fixed. Frozen. Our health and well being, like everything else, was determined by God, or whichever gods were in command at the time. Except for divine intercession, which we might try to invoke, what would be would be. This fatalistic certainty must have been comforting, even though life was "short and brutish." In any case, this phase lasted for millennia until it was disturbed by the appearance and growth of modern science during the Renaissance, which added heat to the system and began to melt the ice.

Science changed not only our now fluid world, but our way of thinking about it. What counted was no longer just what was, but what could be defined, categorized, measured, and enumerated. Macroscopic phenomena could be broken down into their underlying forces and quanta and analyzed.

We began to think not only of nature but of ourselves as complicated, but ultimately understandable, machines. Our conception of disturbances in our well being, of dis-ease, changed from our preordained destiny to a disorder of our body mechanisms, matters of our physics and chemistry. This could, in theory at least, but often in practice as well, be controlled by modifying other underlying or controlling physical or chemical mechanisms. The remarkable success of this new way of thinking acted as a positive feedback system, an amplifying effect. Each new discovery added more heat to the system. It was comforting and comfortable.

In the real world, however, positive feedback loops eventually, inevitably, become controlled by negative feedback of some sort. While we continue to appreciate the advances that scientific medicine has made possible, we are becoming aware of its limits and its unexpected side effects. We are living longer, long enough to suffer more. We are living and dying with hitherto unthought-of and incurable diseases. The heat is getting too intense. We're starting to get uncomfortable.

We are becoming increasingly aware that something difficult to define, something uniquely human, has been missing. We realized that by focusing on the disease, and what we could do about it, we forgot about the people who have the disease and those who love them. By concentrating on the effectiveness and efficiency of the system, we gave undue emphasis to the healers, rather than to those who need healing. Perhaps we need a new renaissance.

It is possible, and there are embryonic signs. We have seen remarkable changes towards patient-focus in some isolated segments of our health care system. In maternity care, for example, a short half-century ago, pregnancy was treated like a disease: pregnant women were treated with intrusive prescriptions and proscriptions and hospitalized for prolonged periods. In labor, they were isolated from loved ones. Massive sedation and general anesthesia excluded them from their awareness of, their involvement in, the birth experience. This is no longer the case. Women wanted more and got it. Now women can once again be awake and aware during the profound, life-changing experience of giving birth. Much of these changes came as a result of women sharing their experiences, making their wishes known, and demanding what they believed was their due.

Something similar is happening towards the end of life. As we recognize that we are increasingly living and dying with long-lasting, incurable diseases, we are beginning to sense the importance of patient autonomy, self-management, home care, and supportive services. The community is starting to be recognized as the wheel of the health system, with the person as its axis.

These budging changes may subside and be squelched by the massive inertia of the system as a whole. The juggernaut we call the health care system may roll on, crushing everything in its path. Or the small changes may accumulate until they reach the tipping point.

Change will come. We can't foresee when or know the direction it will take, but we know it will come. What we can do, however, is try to nudge it in what we think is the right direction.

This book about Sholom Glouberman's operation is such a nudge. It is one person's anecdote, albeit the narrative experience of someone articulate, eloquent, and more knowledgeable than many about all aspects of the health care system. It is a word picture worth a thousand data points. It can give us insights into the depths of our ambivalence to the health care system. If it stimulates others to add their own experiences – neutral, positive, or negative – to the mix, we may find that the health care system is ready for its new birth.

Murray W. Enkin
Alejandro R. Jadad
Toronto, March 2010

Acknowledgments

This book involved many people. There were numerous drafts that attempted to capture the experience of being a patient in a way that might be useful not only to patients themselves, but also to those who care for them and those who think about health and health care. As Murray Enkin and Alex Jadad note in their insightful foreword, the book is part of a larger project. *My Operation* is about my experience, and I must acknowledge those who helped me through it, those who helped me to write about it, and finally those who recognized a wider need to improve the patient experience for everyone.

The people who supported me most during the experience of becoming a patient were my family and close friends whose constant presence, concern, and human warmth shielded me from the most difficult parts of this journey and helped me to maintain hopefulness throughout. My wife Susan rarely left my side – staying over for many nights, always there with loving attentiveness. My son Misha wrote up the reports for family and friends, and our daughter-in-law Margaux Williamson was there to help Misha and Susan. Our friends Jerry and Ruthy Portner came to Toronto especially to be with us during the time of the operation. Berl Schiff accompanied us to the major medical meetings and supported us in the difficult times. His wife Gissa and our friend Chaya

Thalenberg were always available to Susan. Many of our relatives were there for us. Susan's brother Chaim Tannenbaum came to make sure that his sister could go home to shower. His wife Susannah Phillips stayed in touch throughout. My brother Nochem and his wife Dina came to be with us. Our neighbour George Vegh drove me to the hospital during the worst crisis. All our friends and many of our relatives visited and helped: David Berlin, Debbie Kirshner, Meri Collier, Dan Perlitz, Eleanor Enkin, Murray Enkin, Alex Jadad, Shana Pofelis, Ray Brown, Simon Schneiderman, Rafael and Anna Lopez-Corvo, Saul and Annie Levine, Marsha and Steve Herbert, Keith Oatley and Jennie Jenkins, Earl Berger and Joan Moss, Marshall and Sheila Walker, Sylvia Weininger, Patsy Baranek and Tony Doob, Sandy Fainer, Ariadne Fainer-Siotis, Jerry and Sheila Goldenberg, Ryan Kamstra, Sheila Heti, Elise Parker, Marvyn Novick, Alex Tarnopolsky and Alma Petchersky, Ted Ball, Phyllis Platt and Peter Moss, Linda Lipsky and Ed Elkin, Hershey and Esther Frank, Kevin Pask and Marcie Frank and their daughters, Violet and Emma Pask, Hodl Tannenbaum, André Dascal, and Terry Tannenbaum.

There is little doubt that the medical, nursing, and other staff at the hospital saved my life. They also made the experience what it was. Some of the care was outstanding. At the Patients' Association of Canada, we have initiated the Patients' Choice Award for health practitioners who are especially sensitive to patients. In my story, there is a clear winner: A. Zakizewski was a member of the Critical Care Support Team. She was available, humane, and forthcoming in a time of great need. She listened carefully, answered all our questions, and reported faithfully and legibly into the medical record.

The list of names below is not inclusive. It is not complete because some of the names in the medical record were illegible and there were many other people who cared for me whose names I never knew and who are not listed in the record. The number is longer than the list of family and friends.

Acknowledgments

The health practitioners: Dr. Edward Rawling, Surgeon; Dr. Richard Reznick, Surgeon; Dr. Sidney Sussman, Radiologist; Dr. Stuart McCluskey, Anesthesiologist; Dr. Darlene Sherry Fenech, Fellow, Colorectal surgery; Dr. Todd Penner, Minimally Invasive Surgeon; P. Bernard, Registered Practical Nurse; Dr. Ajay K. Sahajpal, Surgical Resident; Helen Thomas, Registered Nurse; A. Zakizewski, Registered Nurse; M. Johnson, Registered Nurse; M. Thomson, Registered Nurse; John Cardella, Registered Nurse; V. White, Registered Nurse; Dr. Martin E. O'Malley, Radiologist; Dr. J. Choi, Chief Surgical Resident; Sonia, Home Care Nurse; Rachelle, Home Care Nurse; Dr. Martin E. Simons, Radiologist; Dr. Zaid Yasser, Surgical Resident; Dr. Manish Taneja, Radiologist; Dr. Khumar Huseynova, Surgical Resident; Dr. David Gianfelice, Radiologist; Dr. B. Basarra, Infectious Diseases Resident; Dr. Marc Allen, Internist; Dr. Mirek Otremba, Internist; Lay Chain Wong, Echocardiography Technician; Beth McCallum, Registered Nurse; Marian Garcia, Registered Practical Nurse; Dr. M. Quteri, Resident; J. Cleary, Registered Nurse; Dr. Adrienne Chan, Infectious Diseases Fellow; Dr. Runjan Chetty, Pathobiologist; Dr. David Carr, Emergency Medicine Physician; Dr. Zeinab Layton, Radiologist; Dr. Joel S. Yaphe, Emergency Medicine Physician.

Support for the book has come from City Life and Well-Being: The Grey Zone of Health and Illness, a project of the Canadian Institutes of Health Research. Alan Blum is the lead investigator; he has encouraged me in word and deed. He sent capable research assistants for the several years that it took to put together the manuscript in its present form. Katie Aubrecht did heroic work while I was still quite disabled after the operation. She transferred much of the medical record from almost illegible handwriting, decoded the abbreviations, prepared the glossary, and reformatted much of the text before she disappeared. Jan Plecash helped to finalize parts of the document, but mostly she provided excellent records of meetings about the patient experience that infuse the book with greater meaning. Ariane Hanemaayer kept a sane hold over the material and reformatted it to prepare the first camera-ready version that allowed us to mock up the book. She also helped to research the new ways to publish independently. The creation of Health and Everything Publications was done with her help. Ryan Devitt meticulously and expertly edited the text and completed the book's design, with help from Roisin Bonner and Paula Blum. Michaela Cornell was also instrumental in the book's launch.

Versions of the book were read by many individuals and at a long-standing book club that my wife and I belong to. It has been discussed with friends and colleagues and presented at meetings of the Patients' Association of Canada. Some of the friends who read the manuscript include Anton and Annabel Obholzer, Jo Ivey Boufford, James Wilk, Keith Oatley, Jennie Jenkins, Patsy Baranek, Morris Moscovitch, Alina Gildner, Debbie Kirshner, Pierre Gerlier Forest, Elke Grenzer, Alex Jadad, and Murray Enkin.

Finally, I would like to acknowledge the people I have talked to about the patient perspective and whose help contributed to the development of the Patients' Association of Canada. They made me understand how this book can be a contribution to understanding and improving the patient experience. They are Eleanor Enkin, Murray Enkin, Alejandro Jadad, Jan Plecash, Larry Enkin, Elke Grenzer, Anita Stern, Ariene Hanemaayer, Amanda Delong, Rosalee Berlin, Elinor Caplan, John Feld, Jonathan Tucker, Kevin Leonard, Laura O'Grady, Bob Lester, Neil Stuart, Steve Herbert, Vytas Mickevicius, Judy Steed, Adrienne Shnier, Aileen O'Dowd, Alan Engelstad, Don Schurman, Frances Slayton, Kathie Busija, Laura Alper, Mark Sarner, Norman Kalant, Ryan Devitt, Sandy Storms, Zal Press, Alan Blum, Brian Goldman, Carol Kitai, Dan Florizone, Dan Perlitz, Dave Clements, James Wilk, Janet Davidson, Jo Ivey Boufford, Marvyn Novick, Normand

Acknowledgments

Rinfret, Phyllis Yaffe, Sheila Damon, Stan Feldman, Tess Weber, Kevin Smith, Michael Decter, Tim Brodhead, Vivek Goel, Ross Upshur, Mimi Lowi, Maureen O'Neil, PG Forest, Kate McGarrigle, David Wiljer, Louise Lemieux Charles, Abe Fuks, Martin Dawes, André Picard, Diane Gagnon, Kevin Barcley, Nick Offord, Peter Moss, Jonathan Guss, Pat Nelson, Suzanne Strasberg, Helen Ferrigan, Jennifer Oosterbaan, Neil Seeman, Viola Desanti, Gar Mahood, Tom Closson, Paul Genest, Stephen Huddart, Ashley Menard, Melissa Wheeler, Elmer Mascarhena, Don Willison, Paul Hebert, Tina Smith, and Pinchas Gutter.

Introduction

My father died young of colon cancer many years ago. He had a horrific death. The cancer had already invaded much of his body when it finally blocked his intestines and was discovered. My mother was there all day, every day, and I would be with him every afternoon and evening for his two long stays at the Royal Victoria Hospital in Montreal. We could see him slowly deteriorate as the cancer spread and stopped his liver from working. He turned into a yellowed skeleton of himself and was in enormous pain that was only slightly dulled by the morphine. Towards the end, he pleaded for death to release him. Finally, he had a massive stroke and became comatose. Though it was known that he would never recover, he was kept alive for more than two weeks. For those weeks, I had to moisten his mouth often so that sores would not form. I still remember the process of pushing his teeth apart and inserting a wet sponge and I can still smell his breath. His death was a release from months of terrible pain. His dying has had a profound influence on how I think about life and death and health and hospitals.

Perhaps because I had spent many weeks there with my father, the Royal Victoria Hospital (RVH) was familiar to me when I began to work there as a consultant planner. I still provide advice and support to senior managers and professionals there, though it has now merged with other hospitals to become the McGill University Health Centre, one of Canada's foremost teaching and research hospitals. The two very different kinds of experiences at the RVH helped me to understand how hospitals work and to engage with doctors, nurses, and all manner of professionals and administrators in the always compelling, often complex, and occasionally frenetic health care world.

I went from the RVH to the King's Fund in London England, a health care think tank, which gave me access to the entire National Health Service. There I consulted across the spectrum of health professionals, hospitals, and other services and designed and directed their flagship management program. Back in Canada, I continued many of these activities. I regularly observe health care on the ground at the Baycrest Centre for Geriatric Care, where I am the Philosopher in Residence, and at other hospitals in the Toronto area. For a number of years, I led the health policy group at the Canadian Policy Research Networks, and I now direct The International Masters Program for Health Leadership at McGill University.

My background has led me to try to make health care better and some of my books and articles have even had some influence on systems in Canada and abroad. My experiences made me feel comfortable everywhere in the health field: I saw myself as a health care insider. I felt confident that when I became a patient, I would be able to handle the system pretty well. How wrong I was!

Colon cancer runs in families and is preventable if caught early enough. When I turned fifty, I began to have regular colonoscopies as is generally recommended, particularly for those with a family history like mine. I had three or four colonoscopies that showed no problems; in 2005, however, they found a polyp that could not be removed with the colonoscope, which meant that I had to see a surgeon.

This was when the problems began. I became a patient and the system took over. My experience, understanding, and sophistication stood for naught. The surgeon examined me and booked me for an operation to have part of my large intestine removed in August of 2005.

The experience of being a patient was dramatically different from what I thought it would be. This very difference surprised me, frightened me, and put me into a state of emotional and physical upheaval that just seems to have ended recently. It was the strength of this experience that led me to record the events of *My Operation* and my reaction to them.

My story is not particularly unusual. I hope that it captures some of what many of us have lived through during and after hospital stays. I hope especially that it retains the flavour of some of the easy and many of the more difficult interactions that patients have with health professionals and hospital staff.

After some effort and with a great deal of help from Sharon Rogers, the patient representative at the University Health Networks (UHN), I managed to obtain a complete copy of my medical record. It helped me verify the detail of what had happened to me. Although I had vivid memories of the experience, I was sure that many of the days had blurred together. At times, I could not tell day from night. The record helped get the dates straight, find out who had actually cared for me, and clean up some of the details. Later, research assistants transcribed and decoded as much of the record as they could, and I have included this material with the narrative as a supplement and at times a contrast to my experience. It is not necessary to read the record to follow the plot, and I have distinguished it from the rest of the text by changing the font size and by inserting a grey background wherever possible. The record acts as a counterpoint to my experience, and those readers who want to can compare my experience on a particular day with the nursing notes, look at the test results, and do some deeper excavations into the detail.

I have included many of the names of people I encountered. The story is not about an anonymous patient. Nor is it a clinical case study. I was the patient, and there is therefore no reason to hide or disguise my name or the names of those who played a part in caring for me. I have sent the book to my surgeon, Dr. Richard Reznick, who had primary responsibility for my care, and I offered to have him join me in editing it for publication and for further corrections. Perhaps understandably, he refused. I have also sent it to both Mary Ferguson-Paré, the Vice President of Professional Affairs and Chief Nurse Executive who is in charge of nursing services at UHN, and to Sharon Rogers. When they made them, I have taken up some of their suggestions for revision. Of course, I assume all responsibility for the inevitable mistakes.

Chapter One

Before the Surgery

April 2001: Colonoscopy, Rudd Clinic

What niggled was the early visit to Dr. Molloy. Colonoscopies were cleanups like Roto-Rooters – very unpleasant but necessary visits to unseen plumbing. Largely forgotten parts had to be inspected and cleaned up occasionally; dangerous detritus had to be identified and cut out to reduce the chance of malignancy.

The clinic, in a large office building, was an efficient public space, buzzing with many women who worked in subservient support of the male physicians. The doctors in white floated in and out of the room only occasionally, spending most of their time in a colon-like unseen maze of corridors beyond the protective counter. The women behind the counter were hooked to telephones and gazed blankly into computer screens.

The Rudd Clinic is one of several institutions dedicated to colonoscopies in Ontario. There is also, for example, the amusingly named Upper Canada Lower Bowel Clinic. These clinics are not in hospitals. In Canada, such clinics are free at the point of delivery to all patients who are referred by their family doctors for a colonoscopy. The government pays a set fee for each colonoscopy performed at the clinic. Often, these clinics are owned by one or a small group of the doctors who work in them. A percentage of the fees paid to individual doctors is used to cover the overhead costs and provide a profit to the owners. But, because the distinction between "private" and "public" care is a confused muddle in Canada, the single source of funding makes many consider them to be part of the public system even though they are privately owned.

Dr. Molloy himself was a crumbly old man. He limped and creaked and fretted and creaked and grumbled as he prepared to insert the tube of the equipment. His new assistant was unsure of herself; I never got her name. It became clear that she didn't know what he wanted, and this, it turned out, was their first encounter with each other. He welcomed her by saying, "You're new, you sure you know what to do?"

The camera at the head of the tube allowed me to watch the proceedings in living colour. A day of purging and fasting had rendered my insides a glowing pink and the tube traveled through my brightly lit colon as if it were in an amusement park tunnel. As the colonoscope approached the far reaches of my innermost being, Dr. Molloy said, "Look there is a polyp! We can snip it out...but it's playing hard to get... move the tube. Now I have it."

I began to think that Dr. Molloy was one of the large number of doctors who continue to practice after their sell-by date. There is no mandatory retirement date for doctors. In the United States, for example, there are more than 1200 doctors who are still practicing after their ninetieth birthday. A large number of them find it hard to stop. Dr. Michael De Bakey, the first man to transplant a human heart, said "I would not mind having a 91 year old surgeon." He said this when he was 91. In Canada in 2007, there were 338 doctors over the age of 80 who were still practicing.

And he snipped.

"That's only a piece of it. Let's get the rest. Oh, you've lost that bit...Let's retrieve it...No, it's gone again. Let's get the rest of it. Here's another piece. We're running out of time. We'll send what we've got to the lab...You need more training...Let's get out. There's no more time..."

To me, "We found a polyp and have got some of it, but a bit is still in there. Come back in three years and we'll see what happens."

"Are you sure that we should wait that long?" I asked.

"I'm sure this thing is not malignant, but there is not enough to send to the lab," he replied. "It's just in a hard place to reach. The part we lost will emerge in the natural course of things."

I was having none of this reassurance from a man who appeared to have lost control of the procedure. The exchange itself was frightening. What was going on? Why was he so pressed for time that he couldn't get it all out? I had the feeling that Dr. Molloy was worried about his own continuing competence and perhaps his place in the clinic. His concerns about being supported by a new nurse and about taking too much time were signs of this.

My friend Ruthy Portner had been misdiagnosed by a doctor at the teaching hospital. He refused to believe that her rectal bleed was anything more than hemorrhoids. She went to see a naturopath for these symptoms and after looking at her, he told her to get to an oncologist as quickly as possible for tests. It turned out that she had rectal cancer. Luckily, she survived, but they had to take out her anal sphincter and close her rectal opening, so she was left with a colostomy and a bag for life. Slight medical misjudgments, as I knew too well, can have disastrous effects.

March 2002: Colonoscopy, Rudd Clinic

A polyp can't grow so quickly, but three years seemed too long for me to wait, so I asked my family doctor to book a colonoscopy for the next year. Dr. Molloy was unavailable, thank god. The new endoscopist, Dr. Edward Rawling, performed the procedure without any of the fuss that had accompanied my previous visit. He found another polyp and excised it. Afterward, he brought me into his small office and told me that the polyp would be sent for analysis and I would get the results in several weeks, but he, like Dr. Molloy, was sure that it was not malignant.

My adventures with the colorectal world then gained a new dimension. I had forgotten to stop my daily aspirin tablet, which helps prevents heart attacks and stroke and is recommended for those of us who are getting on. It also prevents the blood from clotting and so I began to shit blood the next day. At the emergency room, they assured me that there was nothing wrong beyond the results of the colonoscopy. It would go away. And it did. I later learned that the polyp was not malignant: I was cancer free. Now I could put all of this aside for three years until my next colonoscopy.

Winter 2003: Otto Weininger has Colon Cancer

In 2003, my faith in the importance of colonoscopies was reinforced and, if anything, increased. Otto Weininger, a feisty, combative, and wonderful friend in his mid seventies, went for his first colonoscopy and found that he had metastasized colon cancer. This was during the Toronto SARS epidemic in 2003. He spent almost three weeks in hospital for bowel surgery. He was not allowed any visitors and was eventually sent home to die. He quickly deteriorated as the cancer that had spread to his liver and other organs began to kill him. This was not an easy death. When I visited him, I held the hand of a wizened, yellow old man who was filled with morphine to dull the constant pain. He died a few days later.

November 2004 to April 2005: Colonoscopies, Rudd Clinic

I booked a colonoscopy in November 2004. This time, Dr. Rawling found a polyp, which he cut out. As he went further into the colon, he discovered another polyp that was visible but could not be excised. This was more worrisome. He called for another colonoscopy several months later just to see if he could now get it. But the second polyp was stuck to the wall of the colon and was tubulovillous. That meant that it would become malignant in time and would have to be taken out. He looked carefully at this new polyp, which I have come to believe was the remnant of the first polyp that Dr. Molloy had not completely removed. It had grown against the wall of the colon and could not be cut out using the tools available in the colonoscopy. Dr. Rawling referred me to a colorectal surgeon, Richard Reznick.

RUDD CLINIC

Wm. WARREN H RUDD, M.D., FRCS(C), FACS
FOUNDER AND DIRECTOR

J.D. HAMILTON, M.D., FRCS(C)	J.S. LAUGHTON, M.D. FRCS(C), FACS
M.A.P. SMITH, M.D., FRCS, FRCS(ED), FRCS(C)	E. STERNTHAL, M.D., FRCS(C), FACS
A.R. MAHARAJ, M.D., DABS	E.G. RAWLING, M.D., FRCS(C), FACS
D.R. LINDSAY, M.D., FRCS(C)	J.M. FAREKH, M.D. FRCS(E), FRCS(C)
W. ATHERTON, M.D., FRCS(C)	J.P. McKENNA, M.D., FRCS(C)

April 28,2005
Dr. Richard Reznick
Princess Margaret Hospital
Tel: (416) 340-4137
Fax:(416) 340-4211

Dear Dr. Reznick:

RE: MR. SEYMOUR GLOUBERMAN-Chart No. 67608
-OHIPNo, 4433950088 HA

Seymour is gentleman seen on April 28, 2005 with a very sessile polypoid cobblestone type of lesion in the proximal ascending colon just distal to the ileocecal valve which was biopsied and partial snare removal showing tubulovillous adenoma changes which cannot be removed endoscopically but will require surgical consultation.

I have referred him to Dr. Richard Reznick.

He has a very strong family history of colon cancer. Today's pathology will be forthcoming. The initial pathology done on April 01, 2005 is included.

Always sincerely,

Edward G. Rawling, M.D., FRCS(C), FACS
EGR/rm
C.C: Dr. Robert A. Kingstone, 875 Eglington Ave. W., Toronto, ON M6C 3Z9

123 Edward St. Suite 825 Toronto, ON M5G 1E2
E-mail: reception@ruddclinic.com
Phone (416) 597-0997 Fax   (416) 597-2912

Of course, I checked Dr. Reznick out with my more knowledgeable friends, Murray Enkin and Alex Jadad. Alex is a professor in the medical school at the University of Toronto. When he heard that I might have to have surgery, he suggested that he could act as my external medical support person. He would make himself available if there were unanswered questions and if I needed further interventions. He knew Richard Reznick as a colleague. Dr. Reznick was the Professor of Surgery as well as the head of his department. He was interested in education and a careful and kind man according to those who knew him.

While working at the King's Fund in England, I had given a talk to a group of visiting Swedish physicians about my impression of the three classes of patients that doctors in Canada and the UK seemed to have. First-class patients were members of one's family, families of close colleagues, celebrities one wished to please, and other very select individuals. Second-class patients were from one's own middle class – people who shared values and attitudes and had middle-class expectations about such things as appointment times and civil discussion. Third-class patients were not of one's class, often sought primary care in emergency rooms or clinics, were accustomed to waiting in long queues, and often had some trouble communicating. I asked the Swedish doctors whether this distinction was true in Sweden and they began with quiet denials that escalated into a long, loud argument about actual practice in their home country.

Although I was often a first-class patient for the doctors I worked with at the Royal Victoria Hospital, I had no such status at the Toronto General and was clearly a second-class patient for Dr. Reznick. Nor did I want any special privileges beyond those of a second-class patient; it should be enough to get me through.

May 2005: Visit to Dr. Richard Reznick

When I called for an appointment, Dr. Reznick's office told me that it was necessary for me to have an enema before I saw him in case he wanted to do a rectal examination. I thought that it was probably unnecessary given the fact that the polyp was not even close to the rectum.

I thought to myself that I should not do this, this is not for me. Is it merely an assertion of medical authority? What do I know?

But did I prepare for the visit by having an enema? I did...

My wife Susan insisted on accompanying me to all my medical appointments from this time on; she wanted to know what was happening, to ask her own questions, and to relieve her anxiety about my prospects. Dr. Reznick introduced us to his resident, a trainee in surgery. He was a tall, thin, friendly fellow who would do the initial examination. He asked lots of questions about my state of health and especially about the nature of my bowel movements. I was used to this because for years, my mother, as did many other Jewish mothers, had a continued interest in this aspect of my life. Of course, the resident never suggested that I required a rectal examination. Should I have found out more about their requirements? What else should I have asked? Should I merely have been less compliant? Was I a wimp?

Dr. Reznick then came in, smiled, and said that we would do yet another colonoscopy before he would operate. He would be more aggressive than the endoscopist and might be able to excise the growth. He added that if, however, his attempts should perforate the bowel, he would do a surgery immediately. The hospital was right there for emergency surgeries when necessary, but the prospect was nonetheless frightening. The preparation for the colonoscopy was pretty arduous: it was as if I were preparing for colon surgery, so I was required to drink a gallon of Colyte the evening before I went. Colyte was a powder that came in a gallon jug to which one added water. The resulting drink made me mildly nauseous after every glass. It took an hour to get through all of it and resulted in a rapid and complete evacuation of the bowel. This was a much more unpleasant preparation than for other colonoscopies. But since there was the possibility that surgery might be necessary, I could hardly object.

COLONOSCOPY PREPARATION   **Date: 30/05/05**

GOLYTELY/CO-LYTE

Items needed from the Pharmacy:
1. Golytely, Co-lyte or KLEEN-Prep
2. 3 Dulcolax tablets-(3x5mg tablets)

Day Prior to Procedure/Surgery:
8:00 AM Take 3 Dulcolax tablets, and add tap water to the Golytely mixture, following the directions on the package, and chill in the refrigerator.
5:00 PM Begin drinking the Golytely mixture at the rate of one 8 ounce glass every 10 to 20 minutes. Drink the portions rapidly; do not sip it in small amounts. Continue drinking in this manner until the mixture has been consumed. You may use any mouthwash to rinse your mouth between glasses. This helps to cut the salty taste of the mixture. The first bowel movement should occur approximately one hour after you start drinking the mixture. Drink only clear fluids (no milk or citrus juice) until after your procedure.

Procedure Day:
Plan to be at the hospital for approximately 2 hours following your test and arrange for someone to take you home. You will NOT be allowed to drive yourself as you will be having sedation during your test! Bring your Ontario Health Card and your hospital cards with you and come to the 2nd floor Eaton Wing (follow signage Endoscopy/Motiity).

Appointment; Wed. June 1, 2005 please arrive at 8:00a.m.

Wednesday, June 1, 2005: Colonoscopy, Dr. Reznick

My wife Susan once more accompanied me. She feared that I had a deathly case of cancer. She requested the support of another friend, Berl Schiff. The three of us came to the surgical outpatient area very early and were ignored by the people behind the counter. We waited to be called but were not. Well over an hour later, Berl said that I was oddly not proactive here. In fact, I seemed to him to be particularly passive; I should go to the counter and ask about what was going on. I went to the counter and asked. The clerk was not there that day and they had somehow lost track of my presence. I was then quickly assigned to a room and hurriedly given an injection of a drug that would make me very groggy during the colonoscopy. Dr. Reznick came in, smiled, and began the procedure. I remember none of it. I do recall that afterwards he said that he could not extract the growth and would have to do a colon resection. Apparently, he said a lot more to me, but I was half asleep from the pain killer. He also spoke to Susan and Berl and told them much more. We arranged a date for the surgery after my summer vacation. He said that he would perform the surgery laparoscopically and would be assisted by another surgeon who had performed many more such procedures than he had. I was aware that he himself had not usually performed laparoscopic surgery but had usually made larger abdominal incisions. I also knew that it was best not to allow surgeons to learn on you. On the other hand, I understood that recovery from laparoscopic surgery was quicker. But I think that, for the most part, I was his patient and accepted his suggestion that it be done this way.

This acceptance and passivity is quite characteristic of the patient-doctor relationship. Doctors both young and old have told me that their recommendations are almost always accepted by virtually every patient they see. Even when they themselves would like to explore alternatives, the patient will often say, "What do you think I should do, doc?" and accept whatever is suggested. Although there are many explanations for this passivity, this is pretty much standard patient behaviour. Mine was hardly unusual.

CHART COPY

Date: 01/06/05

UNIVERSITY HEALTH NETWORK
Toronto General Hospital
200 Elizabeth Street,
Toronto, Ontario M5G 2C4
Health Records Services
* * * CHART COPY * * *
NAME: Glouberman,Seymour
DOB: 10Octl940 MRN: 239 7544   G
VISIT #: 255018512
LOCATION: Active IP
Date Dictated: 01Jun2005
PROCEDURE: Colonoscopy
DATE OF PROCEDURE: 01June2005
SURGEON: Dr. R. Reznick
ASSISTANT: Dr. F. Quereshy
ANESTHETIST:
ANESTHESIA:
PREOPERATIVE DIAGNOSIS:
POSTOPERATIVE DIAGNOSIS:

CLINICAL NOTE:
This is an operative note on Mr. Seymour Glouberman who underwent a colonoscopy on June 1st, 2005. Mr. Glouberman is a gentleman who was referred to us from the Rudd Clinic by Dr. Rawling who identified a sessile polypoid lesion in the proximal ascending colon on April 28th, 2005. He was referred to us for an assessment regarding surgical options. After a long discussion with the patient in our Outpatient Ambulatory clinic it was decided that we would take him to the Endoscopy Suite for a colonoscopy to evaluate this sessile polyp. After informed consent was obtained the patient was brought to the Endoscopy Suite on June 1st, 2005.

OPERATIVE NOTE:
The patient was brought into the Endoscopy Suite after receiving a bowel preparation. The patient was then positioned in the left lateral decubitus position and 2 mg of VERSED along with 50 mg of DEMEROL were given in divided doses. The colonoscope was then inserted per anus and was advanced through the rectum through the sigmoid, the descending colon, the transverse colon, the ascending colon, and to the cecum. The cecum was identified with its normal anatomical structures including the ileocecal valve. Of note, 5 cm proximal to the ileocecal valve we identified a 4 cm sessile villous tumour. This could not be endoscopically removed and several photographs were taken endoscopically of this lesion. A second

18

CHART COPY CONTINUED

Date: 01/06/05

sessile villous lesion was identified adjacent to this polypoid lesion and was removed using the snare electrocautery. This was then retrieved through suction using the endoscope. The colonoscope was then slowly and gently removed with thorough evaluation of the remainder of the colon.

There were no other tumours or inflammatory changes that were identified through the transverse colon, descending colon, sigmoid colon, or rectum.

The patient tolerated the procedure well. There were no intraoperative complications. The patient was then transferred to PACU in stable condition.

After completing the colonoscopy and identifying this villous tumour 5 cm proximal to the cecum, it was decided that surgical intervention would be the most appropriate treatment option. As such, we have arranged for Mr. Glouberman to undergo a preoperative assessment for a laparoscopic hemicolectomy in the near future. He will be contacting our office in the near future here in the General Surgery Ambulatory Outpatient Clinic.

As always, it is a pleasure participating in the help and care of your patients. If any further questions should arise please feel free to contact us if necessary.

Dictated by: Dr. Fayez A. Quereshy

Service of: Richard K. Reznick, MD, MEd, FRCSC, FACS
Professor of Surgery, University of Toronto
Department of Surgical Oncology
Tel: 416-340-4137
Fax: 416-595-9846

E-mail: richard.reznick@utoronto.ca
cc. Dr. Robert Kingstone, MD
Dr. Richard K. Reznick, MD
Dr. Edward G. Rawling, MD
Dr. Alejandro R. Jadad Bechara, MD

Susan was quite frightened. I was not. It was a rather uneven division of emotional labour in which I had to be the brave one and she could be fearful. I wonder how

19

many couples assume different parts of the worry and stress surrounding such life events. Still, I recognized that I would have to prepare myself for the surgery and recovery. I did lots of looking on the internet about colon resection and found a complete description of the procedure that described how they would go in, what they would do, and what the recovery time should be. Many easily accessible websites have such descriptions.

My cousin, Hodl Tannenbaum, told me that her son-in-law Robert had the procedure when they discovered a growth like mine in his colon. Robert was a strong cyclist and he was back on his bike in a month. I felt reassured and thought that I should build up my capacity to recover by means of a fitness regimen at our neighbourhood pool. I wanted to swim a kilometre at least once a day for the months of June and July. We arranged to visit our friends Shana Pofelis and Ray Brown in San Diego for three weeks in August. But after going to the pool for a few weeks, my shoulder became so stiff that I could no longer swim and so I went for therapeutic massages in late June. The massage seemed to help until I suddenly developed a pain in my knees, and as they puffed up, I had some trouble walking for any distance and I certainly could not swim.

Friday, July 29, 2005: Pre-Admission

I went to the hospital on July 29 for a pre-admission test. I was given a folder of information about how to prepare myself for the surgery and what I was to take to hospital. I underwent a physical examination by some nurses who took a detailed history, drew blood for testing, gave me a cardiogram, took my blood pressure, and sent me for an X-Ray. A doctor came in to inform me that I had very high blood pressure and that my heart had suffered some effects as a result. Although this would not stop the operation, I should see my family doctor.

NURSING NOTES   **Date: 29/07/05**
                                       Time: 10:00

Patient admitted for nursing assessment. No known drug allergies (NKA). No meds except vitamins. Reason for admission Laparotomy (Lap) Right (R) Colon Resection. Patient is relatively healthy but very anxious. Pre and post op instructions given. Patient told to take nothing by mouth (NPO) after midnight and arrive at hospital 2 hours prior to surgery. Patient had many concerns which were addressed. Patient had no questions.

CHEST X-RAY REPORT   **Date: 29/07/05**
                                       Time: 10:51

Chest
Event Time: Fri, 29 Jul 05 1051
Tue, 02 Aug 05 0835
Documented by:
Accession#: 301694247
Read By: Sidney Sussman, MD
Date Dictated: 29Jul2005
Exam Report :
REPORT (VERIFIED 2005/08/02)
CHEST: TWO VIEWS

This examination is correlated with the report of the previous examination. There is mild cardiomegaly. There is mild tortuosity in the aorta and mild calcification in the aortic knob.
The lungs are clear. There is an azygous lobe noted which is a variant of normal. There is no significant abnormality seen in the mediastinum.

IMPRESSION: There is no active parenchymal lung disease seen.
Verified By: Sidney Sussman, MD

My knees were also terrible. I called to see the doctor that afternoon, but he was not there and instead I saw another doctor in his practice who looked at my knees, diagnosed a case of housemaid's knee, and offered me some high-dose ibuprofen. When she took my blood pressure, she was amazed at how high it was and took back the ibuprofen prescription. She looked at my chart and found previous warning of this in the last EKG that my doctor had somehow not noticed. I wondered what else he had missed. She offered to put me on blood pressure pills while I was away in San Diego, but I refused. I did not want to have my holiday tampered with or to worry about side effects of a new medication while there. She said to put ice on the knee as much as I could.

Monday, August 1, 2005: San Diego

Ice for the knees worked. I was grateful for the diagnosis and the treatment plan. We went to San Diego with my knees in ice and with even more ice on the plane as we traveled across the country. I iced my knees for the first few days in San Diego at our friends Shana and Ray's house and the swelling went down. I sat and read, and as my knee improved, I became more and more unhappy. I was not exercising; I was not enjoying the coast. It didn't feel like a holiday to me. I began to pout. Other friends, Saul and Annie Levine, lent us their place for our holiday, and after a few days, we moved and the holiday began in earnest. Saul had arranged for us to have access to a pool at a sports club and we went there every morning and afternoon. The adult pool was quiet and let Susan read while I swam. In the end, I swam a kilometre each morning and afternoon. My knees cleared up in a week and my shoulder got much better over the three weeks we were there. I was arming myself for the surgery. Susan was too. She later spoke about her fears, but at the time, she soldiered on. I felt myself becoming healthier and stronger as the weeks went by and felt ready to face the surgery when we returned.

Sunday, August 21, 2005: Return to Toronto

We had two days in Toronto before the surgery. On Sunday, we went to the Canadian National Exhibition, a Fall Fair, with our son Misha and with Margaux (our daughter-in-law elect). On Monday, we went out for Chinese food and packed for the hospital. I arranged with Misha to e-mail everyone who should know about the surgery with news of what was going on. I sent him a picture of a colon (reproduced below) so that he could show everyone what was being cut out. The list grew as we went along, and by the time I finally left for the hospital, there were more than twenty on the list, including friends and colleagues of mine and of Misha's.

The piece of colon that was to be removed was a part of the ascending colon close to the cecum.

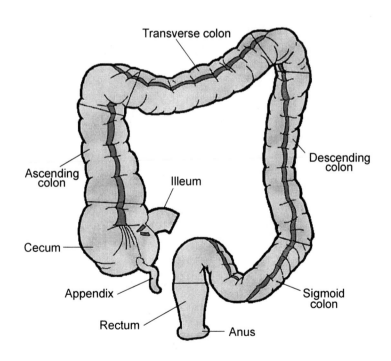

Hi,

As many of you know, my father is scheduled for surgery tomorrow morning, Tuesday Aug 23. The surgery's scheduled for 8:00 a.m. at Toronto General Hospital.

They'll be removing a part of the colon that has a benign polyp, as a purely preventative measure. The procedure will be performed laparoscopically, which means it's minimally invasive, with a number of small incisions rather than one large one.

He will need to stay in hospital while he heals and until his colon starts working again. This stay could last from a couple of days to about week. After that, he'll be at home taking a few weeks off from work as his recovery continues.

My father thought it might be useful to send you all a picture of a colon, and is fond of the one included with this email. I've also included links to information about the procedure.

We'll all be at the hospital on Tuesday, and I'll send an email with news when I can get to an email client, hopefully by Tuesday afternoon.

I'm happy to pass on any notes or messages to my father while he's in the hospital. Just email them to me at this address.

- Misha

Information on Polyps: http://digestive.niddk.nih.gov/ddiseases/pubs/colonpolyps_ez/

Information on Colon Surgery: http://mhriweb.org/patient_information/patient_education/colon_surgery_CONTAINER.htm

On Laparoscopic Colon Surgery: http://www.lapsurg.org/colon.

We were surrounded by friends and relatives. Ruthy and Gerry Portner, our oldest friends, came from Montreal to be with Susan and me at the hospital. Ruthy had had rectal cancer and later a bowel resection and a colostomy. She knew what to expect and would be vigilant in the hospital and lend support to Susan. We both felt lucky to have such very close friends who would travel to be with us now.

Chapter Two

My Operation:
First Hospital Stay

Tuesday, August 23, 2005: My Operation

CLINICAL NOTES
Date: 23/08/05
Time: 7:15-7:30

Admitted ambulatory with wife, pre-op check in.
Patient seen in Pre-Operative Care Unit (POCU).
Chest Checked. Signature Illegible.
60 year old male Post Lap Hemicolectomy
Blood pressure (BP) up – left ventricular hypertro-
phy (LVH). No known allergies (NKA). Normal renal
function.
Plan: Patient-controlled analgesia (PCA) and Toradol
Signed: Acute Pain Service (APS) McCluskey

OPERATING ROOM NOTE
Date: 23/08/05

Reznick/ Penner/ Fenech
Laparoscopic Assisted Right Hemicolectomy.
No complications for cecal polyp.
Signed: Dr. Fenech

On the day of the surgery, August 23, 2005, Berl Schiff joined the four of us in the early morning. We took a taxi to the hospital and went into the admissions area where we waited. Once I went in, they were joined by Misha and Margaux and other friends, Rafael and Anna Lopez-Corvo. Later still, other friends came and went as they waited for my emergence from the operating theatre and the recovery room.

I had learned that John Cleese was having a colon resection at the same time and that he had agreed with his "very nice" surgeon to put the cut-out piece of colon up for auction on eBay after the deed was done. I wondered if I could do the same with my very nice surgeon. I mentioned this to the admitting nurse, but she did not find it funny. I left my bag and was brought into a room where I undressed and put on the patient's uniform of a backless gown. A man came in carrying a small disposable razor and asked to shave the area on my stomach for the surgery. I was then brought into the operating room, this time on a stretcher. Dr. Reznick was there and he introduced me to the anesthetist. He then told me that the surgeon he had asked to assist him would not be available but that another experienced laparoscopy surgeon would take his place.

This was a critical moment. It did not occur to me to defer the surgery at this point or to question the substitution. Later, it became a point of discussion with many friends who claimed that they would have never agreed to this. They would have asked for a non-laparoscopic operation or for a delay. So much for hindsight...I agreed to go ahead. I had come this far and it felt as if there was no turning back. I also now believe that my decision was part of a "dependent patient" way of thinking. I don't remember meeting the substitute surgeon, who was apparently a Dr. Todd Penner.

I recognize that I was not behaving like a cognizant consumer. But I think that patients are not really "consumers." For the most part, we are not shopping for a particular product or service. When we are at the point of treatment, we are usually in no condition to behave like ordinary consumers. We don't pick and choose and take time to try things on. Even if we are not so ill, we want someone who will take care of us and respond to our needs. In these circumstances, it is easy not only to become dependent, but also to hand over much of our decision-making to people we trust. And doctors are professionally meant to be such trustworthy people. We want them to be there for us when we are ill, not only because they know more about such things than we do, but also because they can and do assume a big part of the responsibility for our health since we are too anxious or too sick to do so ourselves.

Now that I was on my back in the operating room, I could look around. The room seemed very large. The anesthetist sat at a table several yards away. Two other women in the room were not introduced (I guess they were operating room nurses). I had been given some kind of injections and fell asleep almost immediately. The surgery proceeded. Happily, I do not remember any of it. The anesthetic was successful.

Date: 23/08/05

OR PROCEDURE NOTES

NAME: Glouberman,Seymour
DOB: 10 October l940
MRN: 239 7544G
VISIT #: 251010054
LOCATION: Active IP
Date Dictated: 23 August 2005
PROCEDURE: Laparoscopic Right Hemicolectomy
DATE OF PROCEDURE: 23 August 2005
SURGEON: Dr. R. K. Reznick
ASSISTANT: Dr. T. Penner
Dr. D. S. Fenech
ANESTHETIST:
ANESTHESIA:
PREOPERATIVE DIAGNOSIS: Villous tumour right colon
POSTOPERATIVE DIAGNOSIS: Same

CLINICAL NOTE: This gentleman has a family history of colon cancer. He had an endoscopy, which revealed a cecal lesion.

OPERATIVE NOTE: With the patient in a lithotomy position the abdomen was appropriately prepped and draped. A vertical midline incision was used to introduce the Hassan insufflator into the abdomen. Three ports, two 5 mm and one 12 mm, were inserted into the abdomen under direct vision. The area over the ileocolic vessels was incised and these vessels were isolated and taken between a vascular stapler. The lateral peritoneal attachments of the cecum and right colon were then divided. The omentum was then lifted antegrade and dissection was continued on the superior aspect of the transverse colon at the hepatic flexure area working around the hepatic flexure and, hence, mobilizing this organ. After sufficient mobility

PROCEDURE NOTES CONTINUED

was created, the midline abdominal incision was enlarged so as to remove the specimen. This was done and a few additional mesenterric vessels were taken between ties. The two ends were divided making sure to have excellent vascularization of the distal segment. A functional end-to-end anastomosis was performed using the GIA apparatus and the TA 55 apparatus. The area was returned into the abdomen and the wounds were closed in layers.
The patient tolerated the procedure well.
Report Type: OR Procedure/Notes
Date Released: 20 February 2006
Date Transcribed: 23 August 2005
Transcribed By: AW
Verification Status: Complete
CC   Dr. Robert Kingstone, MD
       Dr. To Patient Unknown, MD
       Dr. Richard K. Reznick, MD
       Dr. Edward G. Rawling, MD
       Dr. Todd Patrick Penner, MD
       Dr. Darlene Sherry Fenech, MD

Date: 23/08/05
Time: 12:55

NURSING NOTES

Patient arrived to floor from Patient Acute Care Unit (PACU). Patient asleep, raised easily and oriented. Vital Signs (VS): Temperature (T) 36 degrees, Respiration (R) 18, Pulse (P) 53, Blood Pressure (BP)160/60, 4 Litres (L) of oxygen via Nasal Prongs (NP). Chest clear and audible.
Faint bowel sounds present. Abdomen soft and slightly distended, no flatus, steri-strips x 4.
Inferior medial slightly oozy, serous sanguineous, dressing applied. Continue to monitor.
Foley catheter in situ draining clear amber urine, peripheral pulses present (ppp), no edema. Peripheral Intravenous (PIV) infusing lactated ringer's solution (LR). Normal saline (NS) at 125 c/hr, y-connected to patient controlled anesthesia (PCA) morphine.
Stated pain 7/10 in abdomen. Encouraged use.
Patient denies any nausea or pruritus, or dizziness.
No signs of shortness of breath (SOB) or chest pain (CP) noted.
Patient resting in bed.

Signature Illegible

| NURSING NOTES | **Date: 23/08/05**
Time: 13:30 |

Post op bath given, repositioned in bed. Mouth care given. No voiced complaints at this time.
Signed: P. Bernard RPN

| DOCTOR'S ORDER SHEET | **Date: 23/08/05**
Time: 16:05 |

Physician's Order. Versed 2mg and Demerol 50 mg Intravenous (IV) given.
Signed: Dr. Reznick.

I woke up in the recovery room but do not remember much until I was in my own room. Eileen Thalenberg, another friend, appeared, but Susan, Misha and Margaux, Jerry and Ruthy, and Berl and Gissa Schiff were not there. "Where is everyone?" she asked.

"I was wondering the same thing myself," I said, thinking that I must have fallen asleep and missed them.

She went off and eventually found them in the surgery waiting room; they had not been told that I had been transferred to my room even though Susan had asked several times about the transfer. They were wondering why I was so long in the recovery room.

Confused communication recurred at various moments throughout my time in the hospital. Contact with the system was often couched in anxiety, and there were lapses of communication coupled with caring concern almost every day. This kind of anxiety affects all health care workers as well as patients and their families. My friend Anton Obholzer calls it "pixie dust." He says that it emanates from the pain, illness, anxiety, and death that pervade many areas of health care. Because it is difficult to talk about, health care workers are often not aware of their response to it. Lapses in communication are probably one aspect of this kind of pixie dust. They are hardly a result of ill will, but perhaps of an unconscious desire to stay away from the more overt anxiety of patients and those close to them.

CLINICAL NOTES **Date: 23/08/05**
Time: 16:45

At 15:45 patient complained of feeling weak/dizziness. Patient reassessed and Vital Signs (VS) taken. Blood Pressure (BP) 130/70, Oxygen Saturation 98% 3Litres (L) via Nasal Prongs (NP), Pulse (P) 50, Temperature (T) 36, Respiratory (R) 18. Now patient resting and voiced no complaints.

Hello All,
I'm in the hospital now, as I write this, around 3:30 on Tuesday afternoon (may not be able to send for a while) with my mother, Margaux, and Ruth and Gerry Portner. My father's asleep and recovering from the anesthesia and has a little less colon than he did before.
Everything went really well. Everyone was okay handling the stress of the situation. The hospital staff were really helpful and supportive.
Most important, the surgery seems to have gone exactly as planned: They were able to complete the procedure laparoscopically without any trouble or complication. The polyp was fairly big and also fairly superficial. All indications so far are that it is benign, but to confirm this the polyp and surrounding tissue need to be sent to the lab for a biopsy, which should take a week or a little more.
If you want to visit or get in touch over the next few days, the phone number in the room is 416 340 3131 ext. 7149. The room is on the 8th floor of the Eaton Building in Toronto General Hospital, rm 422.
 - Misha

Lots of people had arrived to greet me there by this time. And now everyone was there. I could hold forth; I told everyone how well I was – not in terrible pain, even though I had some trouble moving. For several hours, I drifted between waking and sleeping.

A nurse asked me to try to sit up, but as soon as I did, I began to feel quite light-headed and said that I thought that I would faint if I did not lie down. I was eased back down but I soon felt faint again. A period of fainting and waking now began, and there was a growing concern that all was not well. What could be causing these faints?

I was surrounded by surgical residents who came in and out of my consciousness as I fainted and revived. Dr. Sahajpal, a young man with a street-wise swagger, a knowing manner, and greased, slicked-back hair, confused me with another bearded man, "How ya doin? Why doncha stop causing us all this trouble and quit fainting or we'll have to send you back to the street."

"I'm his wife," said Susan. "What is going on?"

"He has no wife," said Dr. Sahajpal with great confidence while looking at the wrong chart.

"I think you are confusing him with someone else," said my wife.

"I just want him to stop fainting," said Dr. Sahajpal.

They asked me if I had a history of fainting, and I admitted that I did. I had fainted when I was a teenager in synagogue where it became very stuffy. I fainted again several times when I was excessively tired or ill. In fact, I had had a fainting spell several months before when visiting a friend in England at the beginning of a kind of flu. This settled it for some that I was a fainter. It might be that this was my idiosyncratic response to surgery. I might be "just a fainter." This would be my problem, but nothing to concern them.

There has been much discussion about medical reasoning in the last few years. The reasoning in my case is a good example of it. It works most of the time but not always. It is much like the reasoning used by the police: find a plausible suspect as a solution to the case and stay with the suspected solution until you get a conviction or it is disproved. Coming to a decision and acting on it are the main priorities. If I was a fainter, then the residents would stay with that unless and until it was disproved – nothing to really worry about.

I once wrote a widely read paper with my colleague, Henry Mintzberg, in which we distinguished the culture of doctors from that of nurses and others in the health field. We pointed out that doctors are "interventionists." In hospitals, when doctors see patients during their rounds, they make a decision about what to do next within minutes and move on to the next patient. To some extent, this is because doctors are trained to be very careful managers of their time, which they must mete out to many acutely ill patients. Recently, this approach has been criticized, most eloquently by Jerome Groopman, who argues that doctors are not thoughtful enough and their way of thinking does not respond to the growing appreciation of the chronic and complex nature of most conditions. Treating an acute episode while considering it in the context of a larger, more complex picture is becoming necessary. More thought and fewer quick decisions is, according to Groopman, a better way to proceed in many circumstances. In my case, it would have improved the situation to consider many possibilities other than the fact that I was a "fainter." We seemed not to be privy to any of the deliberations about any alternatives. The possibility that the reconnected colon was still bleeding was not mentioned.

Tuesday, August 23, 2005: Evening

RESPIRATORY THERAPY NOTE	Date: 23/08/05 Time: 20:20

Arterial Blood Gas Analysis (ABG) done from right radial artery, after modified Allen's Test positive. Pressure applied to puncture site. No complications. Patient on oxygen 4 Litres (L) via Nasal Prongs (NP).
Signature Illegible

NURSING NOTES

Date: 23/08/05
Time: 21:10

Received patient at 19:55, alert and oriented x 3 with family members present at bedside. At 20:00 patient stated "I feel like I am going to faint." Patient's eyes rolled back and became unresponsive and code called. Patient then became responsive after a few seconds when shaken by holding patient's shoulders. Dr. Reznick and Dr. Sahajpal up on visit with code team at 20:05 but patient now responsive. Code cancelled – Dr. Reznick at bedside and patient complains of having chest pain. Patient denies pain radiation to neck, arms or jaws. Denies nausea. Patient states chest pain feels like heartburn. Electro cardiogram (ECG) and Troponin (test) ordered by Dr. Reznick. Arterial Blood Gas Analysis (ABGS) done. See vital signs (VS) records for VS and patient transferred to Step Down Unit.
Signed: Helen Thomas
Date: 23/08/05
Time: 21:40
Late entry - bowel sounds (BS) drawn at 20:15 7.1.
Signed: Helen Thomas

Throughout the night, fainting spells recurred every ten to fifteen minutes and I was not getting any better. The surgery team called for support from others. After one fainting spell, they thought that I might have had a heart attack, and when my eyes rolled up into my head, they called a Code Blue for a cardiac arrest and the cardiac team came scrambling. Even though I had not had a heart attack, my heart had not stopped, and the Code Blue was probably unnecessary, they attached a heart monitor to me and transferred me from my room to a high intensity step-down unit on the same floor. They called for the portable X-Ray machine as well.

Late that night Susan called Mary Ferguson Paré and asked if it was okay to call Dr. Reznick at home to tell him about my fainting spells. She encouraged Susan to do it. He said that he appreciated the call, that he would get in touch with the residents to learn more, and that he himself would be in first thing in the morning.

Now I was surrounded by other doctors: young residents, inured to the hospital scene, who were intelligent, well intentioned, yet somehow not quite in charge because the surgeon himself, though appearing only occasionally, was clearly the boss. Other residents also visited. I am not sure who they were, but they came when I was fainting – were they specialists in blood, heart, internal medicine?

I later learned that one of them who I found particularly comforting was not a resident at all but a member of the "Critical Care Outreach Team." Her name is A. Zakizewski, and she is a nurse, not a doctor. She and other members of the team returned often to see how I was, to find out more about how I felt, and to talk to me about what had happened. There was an eagerness and freshness to them. I found out later that they were part of a pilot project.

CRITICAL CARE OUTREACH   **Date: 23/08/05**

Critical Care Outreach – The Critical Care Outreach Pilot project is a systematic approach to the early identification and facilitation of resuscitation of inpatients at risk of deterioration. The purpose of the program is to provide comprehensive critical care services, to provide critical care education to nursing and house staff, and to support and coordinate the care of patients. The participating institutions include TGH, Ottawa Hospital, Oakville Trafalger Hospital, and Queensway Carlton Hospital. The goal of the CCOT is to provide early recognition of patients at risk, adequate aggressive resuscitation and to improve follow-up of patients discharged from ICU.

CCOT CONSULT   **Date: 23/08/05**
                             Time: 21:30-23:30

On arrival: Blood pressure (BP)137/66, Heart Rate (HR) 61 beats per minute (bpm), Oxygen Saturation 98% on 36, Respiratory Rate (RR) 14 364
At 16:12
113:11.1:161

CCOT CONSULT CONTINUED

Date: 23/08/05
Time: 21:30-23:30

Critical Care Outreach Team (CCOT) initial consult for this 64 year old gentleman admitted to general surgery for a lap with right hemicolectomy performed today for excision of polypoid lesion.

History: previous smoker who quit 20 years ago, Tonsillectomy and Adenoidectomy (T&A) performed when patient was a child, kidney stones 25 years ago. No Known Allergies (NKA).

Neurological (Neuro): Called to unit for sudden drop in blood pressure (BP) 76/38 and patient fainted, diaphoretic (excessive perspiration), "unconscious for a few seconds." Complained of feeling dizzy shortly before this. Glasgow Coma Scale (GCS) 15/15, patient drowsy, follows directions well. Pupils equal, react to light (PERL) 2+ mm – no obvious deficits, moves well with normal (N) strength, complained of "mild" epigastric pain. Arterial Blood Gas (ABG) @ 20:31 43/39/117/26/99, respiration non-laboured.

Respiratory (R): Respiratory Rate (RR) = 14 on 3 Litres (L) of oxygen via Nasal Prongs (NP), Saturation (Sat) 98%, chest sounds clear to upper lobes drop to bases slightly. Chest x-ray (CxR) done.

Cardiovascular (CVS): General surgery Dr. Apujazia to review. Afebrile at 36.4 Celsius, oral, cardiomyopathy (CM) in lead II: sinus rhythm (SR) @ 61 beats per minute (bpm). 12 lead, ECG shows normal sinus rhythm (NSR) at 72 bpm, jugular venous pulse (JVP) = 2-3cm.

Gastro-Intestinal (GI): Peripheral pulses present (ppp) x 4 – strong, capillary refill brisk, no edema at present. Right hand peripheral intravenous (PIV) @ 125cc/hr of normal saline solution (NSS). Site in tact, Troponin test negative (-) at 20:30, plan to repeat, blood test (CK) pending.

Genitourinary (GU): BP 137/66, patient lying supine. No diaphoresis at present. Bowel sounds (BS) present today. Abdomen appears soft and rounded. Lap sites dry with scant old blood beneath steri-strip. Urinary Output (U/O) = 142 cc in last 3 hours. Plan to assess every (Q) 2hours. Fluid bolus of 500cc NSS started as per Dr. Apujazia. Then after, 125cc in, discharged as patient awake, BP 140/72 and without nausea. Maintenance drop (gtt) continues.

Spoke with patient's family (son and wife) both report patient has had fainting episodes in past. Most recently this May while away in London. Has had other episodes in past which wife reports coincide with times of stress and exhaustion in the patient's life.

CCOT CONSULT CONTINUED	Date: 23/08/05 Time: 21:30-23:30

No investigations have been done with regard to these incidents. Spoke with Critical Care Outreach Team (CCOT) doctor on call, Dr. W. Casser Denoje, who in turn suggested cardiology consult. Dr. Apujazia paged cardiology who, after referring to fellow, suggested patient required a medical Intensive Care Unit (ICU) consult. ICU resident paged and informed of this patient. Plans to come and assess patient "within next 15 minutes".
Suggested: Complete blood cell Count (CBC) repeated. Troponin reassessment @ 04:30 and 12.30. Bone and mineral profile and electrolytes sent. Urine electrolytes sent. ICU assessment pending.
Thank you for calling CCOT
Signed: A. Zakizewski RN

GENERAL SURGERY NOTES	Date: 23/08/05 Time: 23:30

Patient had fainted at around 20:00 for a few seconds. He mentioned he had chest pain. We did arterial blood gas analysis (ABG), chest x-ray (CxR), electro cardiograph (ECG), cardiac enzyme ek4 Troponin, and all investigations were within normal range. After the patient moved to Medical Surgical Intensive Care (MSIC), or Step Down Unit, he had another episode of fainting. ECG was done again, 500cc bolus was given and the vital signs came back to normal range. ICU consultation to assess the multiple fainting episodes. ECG monitoring. Close observation of vital signs. Repeat complete blood cell count (CBC), Troponin, CxR, ECG.

NURSING ASSESSMENT	Date: 23/08/05

Name: Glouberman
MRN#: 2397544
Neurological/Psychosocial: Awake; eyes closed.
Opened eyes spontaneously to verbal stimuli; obeys commands. Fully oriented and moving all limbs spontaneously and to command.
Oxygen Sat 100%. Plan to titrate it according to Oxygen Saturation. Audible air entry (A/E) to both lung fields.

NURSING ASSESSMENT CONT'D   **Date: 23/08/05**

Cardiovascular: Heart Rate (HR) 6 x regular. Right peripheral intravenous (PIV) normal saline (N/S) 125cc/hr 75cc TBA. Peripheral pulse present (ppp) up to new bag. Brisk capillary refill.
Gastro-Intestinal: Abdomen soft and distended. Bowel sound and passing can be heard even when listening to the lungs.
Genitourinary: Foley – urometer. Dark amber urine.
Signature Illegible

The next afternoon Misha sent out the following:

Hello,
  After the surgery, my father had a couple of fainting spells. These don't seem to be cause for concern – he has a long history of fainting under conditions of stress and exhaustion, but the spells continued through the night, and left him still a little exhausted. Hospital staff are giving him tremendous attention and care, and investigating every last possibility that these fainting spells might relate to.
  I suspect he'll be too tired for visitors for the rest of today (Wednesday), but will likely be better on Thursday. I'll keep you posted.
  We've received tons of emails with regards, wishes, and more colon-related puns than one might expect. Thanks very much – I'm printing up all your messages and passing them on to my father.
      - Misha

I asked him to send a more detailed message to my medical support team.

August 23 2005 Misha to Alex and Murray,
  My father wanted you guys to get the more detailed version of the fainting story: After surgery, he felt faint periodically. At one point, during an examination by a nurse, he complained he was feeling faint, and also that his chest hurt a little. Then he fainted. The nurse, seeing a patient complaining of chest pains

and then having his eyes roll back, immediately called a code blue. She called it off in under a minute, I think, as my father woke up again, but the barrage of machines and bells and people running in and out lasted several minutes.

After this, they moved my father into a room closer to the nursing desk, to monitor him more closely, and also to hook him up for telemetry. They did a number of tests to see whether there was any reason to suspect a heart attack, and they all came back negative. The barrage of the code blue emergency and the subsequent discussion of the possibility of heart trouble was pretty terrifying for my mother, but she pulled through it okay.

My father continued to have fainting spells through the night last night. They're accompanied by sweating and a drop in blood pressure.

While he's generally remarkably stoical about the trials and pains of surgery, I think he finds the fainting spells very very unpleasant.

This morning they found that his hemoglobin was low which would of course contribute to his fainting. They gave him a blood transfusion, and things seem to be much better now. All his signs are okay. He hasn't fainted during the day today at all, although he did have feelings of faintness while the nurses helped him try to sit up for the first time.

He has a long history of fainting when he was a child, and in adulthood he still has occasional moments of feeling faint. And on rare occasions he does faint, generally during experience of stress and/or exhaustion.

Anyhow.

It seems by far the most likely thing is that my father's someone who's a little prone to fainting when tired or stressed and so, in post-operative state, is fainting. Doctors are looking into possible cardiac problems, or the possibility of low hemoglobin due to excess fluid, or the possibility of bleeding during or after the surgery. But mostly all seems okay. He had a rough night, but is in good spirits today, and is receiving fantastic care from hospital staff and great support from friends and family.

   - Misha

Wednesday, August 24, 2005

Tests began to come back: my hemoglobin count was low and falling. I continued to have fainting spells, but now they could do something. They suggested a blood transfusion to raise my hemoglobin levels: I might have some internal bleeding and the transfusion would help. Although I was scared of a transfusion, there seemed little choice. They gave me two units of blood, but my hemoglobin rose and then fell after each transfusion. After I received a third unit, the hemoglobin stayed up.

MSICU CONSULT   **Date: 24/08/05**
                                        Time: 00:50

Medical Surgical Intensive Care Unit (MSICU) – Resident on call

64 year old man with colon cancer surgical procedure (S/P) Laparoscopic Right Hemicolectomy. Referred to ICU due to episodes of hypertension and fainting spells. Patient also had some episodes 3 times before due to stress. Last time was in May. No history of arrhythmia or chest pain.

Past Medical History (P.M.H.):
- Hypertension diagnosis (Dx) untreated. Not given prescription. Ex-smoker.
-Prescription (Rx): Aspirin (ASA) stopped a week ago. Blood pressure (BP) 130/50, Heart Rate (HR) 60, Oxygen Saturation 100%. S1+S2+O. (Note Illegible). Chest clear with good equal breath sound.

Investigation:
- Electro Cardiograph (ECG) – left ventricular hypertrophy (LVH) by voltage
- Chest x-ray (CxR) – cardiomegaly.
- Complete blood cell count (CBC) – Hemoglobin (Hb): 105
- Troponin: less than 0.2

Impression: 64 year old gentleman with fainting episodes and hypotension episode. Most likely due to arrhymic vs vasovagal.

Suggestions:
1) Telemetry monitoring for R. patient.
2) Do magnesium (Mg), phosphate (PO4), calcium (Ca), potassium (K), chloride (Cl), and white blood cell count (WBC) "done".
3) Ringer's Lactate (RL) 1000ml intravenous (IV) bolus.
4) Troponin test 08:00 x 3.
5) Correct electrolytes if present.

Signature Illegible

CCOT CONSULT

Date: 24/08/05

Critical Care Outreach Team (CCOT) follow-up (F/U): Magnesium (Mg) 0.68. Suggested Mg be supplemented. General surgery to please order and Registered Nurse (RN) plans to page.
Troponin, B 12 Mineral, complete blood count (CBC), coagulation and albumin tests. Electrolytes repeated and lactate level results pending. Telemetry reports no ectopy since connection.
Patient was connected to telemetry @ 02:15 and RN reports three more spells where patient complained of dizziness. Hypotensive with two of those spells. He complained of right side chest pain. RN reports patient has been feeling this for a few hours. Pain 1/10.

Thank you – A. Zakizewski

GENERAL SURGERY NOTES

Date: 24/08/05

Blood Pressure (BP) 160/80, Heart Rate (HR) 100, Temperature (T) 37 degrees. Hemoglobin (Hgb/Hb) 85 in the a.m. Multiple syncopal episodes and chest pain. All investigations negative, Troponin test negative. On Examination (O/E): Patient in no acute distress. Abdomen soft, non-tender. Puncture site clear, dry and intact. 2 units packed red blood cells (PRBC).

Signature Illegible

GENERAL SURGERY NOTES

Date: 24/08/05
Time: 08:00

Hemoglobin (Hb) 136 – 84 on Post Operative Day (POD) #1. Patient complained of chest pain (CP)/ syncope. During syncopal episodes blood pressure (BP) down, heart rate (HR) up. Urinary Output (U/O) borderline at 30cc/hr. Stool, no blood. Monitor closely.

(Largely Illegible.)

CLINICAL NOTES   **Date: 24/08/05**

Postoperative Day (POD) #1
Laparoscopic Assisted Right Hemicolectomy
Summary of events overnight (History [Hx] according
to patient and wife):
Patient well post op
Hemoglobin (Hb) checked by junior resident on call,
post op 113
Over the evening several fainting episodes and chest
pain (CP)
Cardiology and Intensive Care Unit (ICU) called; no
cardiac cause
Serial Hb's checked: latest 06:00 = 84
Currently being transferred and feeling much better
Vital signs (VS) overnight (O/N):
Heart rate (HR) max 100 @ 06:00 and midnight – oth-
erwise 50-70
Blood pressure (BP) 140/70 – except fainting epi-
sodes 90/50
Urine output (UO) = 25-40cc/hr
Fluids:
21:00 1500cc bolus normal saline (NS)
23:25 500cc bolus
04:30 1L bolus
06:00 – Hb 84 after 3 L fluids
Now:
Feeling much better
On Examination (O/E): Heart Rate (HR) 87/374, Blood
Pressure (BP) 165/76, Respiratory Rate (RR) 20.
Bruising is mild, no hematoma. Abdomen soft and
non-distended.
Impression: Several syncopal episodes post lap and
Hemicolectomy.
HR down 84 @ 06:00 overnight after 3 L normal
saline (NS) bolus.
Differential diagnosis (DDx): Post op bleed? Vasova-
gal episode?
PLAN:
2 units of blood currently transfusing.
Repeat complete blood cell count (CBC).
Monitor carefully.

Signed: Dr. Fenech / fellow (416-664-0300)

I now had an IV with saline, antibiotics, and blood. I was
also hooked up to a heart monitor and a morphine pump
that allowed me to control the amount of pain killer I took. I

had oxygen coming in through two little pipes that attached to my nose. I had a catheter which took away my urine. I was visited by the cluster of surgical residents, and others with an interest in some aspect of my case seemed also to drop by.

I was given a little plastic toy that I was to blow into and lift the ball. It was nothing less that an "incentive spirometer." It exercised my lungs. Susan felt that this was a very important aspect of my recovery and I was to work at it constantly for the next weeks. It would improve my lung capacity and avert pneumonia. I was both amused and annoyed by it. It is now deep in a bedside drawer, and I still come upon it occasionally when looking for a t-shirt. Am I, in my usual way, saving it for a grandchild to blow the ball into the air?

CCOT CONSULT

Date: 24/08/05
Time: 10:10

Critical Care Outreach Team (CCOT) follow-up (F/U) post overnight (O/N) consult. 64 year old Post Operative Day (POD) #1 for Laparoscopy with Right Hemicolectomy for excision of polypoid lesion. History (Hx) – kidney stones, previous smoker.

SUBJECTIVE (S):
Patient supine, resting and no distress, oriented, calm and no complaint of pain. Verbalizing needs well. Moving well, complained of fatigue. Wife and son with patient.

OBJECTIVE (O):
Neurology (Neuro): Had one additional "fainting episode" @ 07:30 a.m. Placed in trendelenburg position, oxygen increased to 4 Litres (L). Remains conscious during episodes. 1 L normal saline (NS) bolus started and no blood pressure (BP) documented at the time. Presently oriented, alert, no anxiety and no complaint of chest or surgical pain.
Cardiovascular (CV): BP up 184/80, Heart Rate (HR) 92 on telemetry. Telemetry report @ 09:30 normal sinus rhythm (NSR) with occasional premature ventricular beats (PVC). Latest Hemoglobin (Hbg) 06:00 down 84 from 113. 1 unit packed cells (p/c) infusions out of 2 units ordered and no overt bleeding noted.
Patient had one bowel movement (BM) with no melena (blood). HR up, max 100 normally 60-70. Received total 3Litres (L) NS bolus overnight. BP during

44

| CCOT CONSULT CONTINUED | **Date: 24/08/05**
Time: 10:10 |

"fainting episodes" down 90/50. Patient's temperature up 37.7 degrees during p/c infusion. White Blood Cell Count (WBC) 84, Troponin negative.
Respiratory (R): Using oxygen 2 L via Nasal Prongs (NP), Respiratory Rate (RR) 22, Oxygen Saturation 97%. Trachea midline, illegible, patient in no acute distress. Air Entry (A/E) illegible. No chest x-ray (CxR) ordered, able to cough but no sputum.
Gastrointestinal (G.I.): abdomen soft, some bruising midline. BM but no bleeding.
Genitourinary (G.U.): Foley in situ (volume 2375/24hr period). Lasix draining 10 mg intravenous (IV) 11 2 units packed cells (p/c).
Plan:
- Monitor complete blood cell count (CBC) every three hours (q3h) and post 2 units p.c.
- Monitor syncopal episodes and hemodynamics
- Monitor serial troponins
- Monitor fluid status input/output (I/O) over 24 hours
- Continue with telemetry
Will follow – CCOT 416-790-9969

Signed: A. Zakizewski

I was told that I would remain in hospital until my digestive system began to work again, and so one of the nurses' tasks was to listen to my stomach for the sounds of digestion. Passing gas would be another sign of the reawakening of my digestive tract. Any turn or sudden movement caused quite a lot of pain, so I had to lie on my back and could only roll over to my side after quite a while. I found that I could make myself more comfortable by adjusting the bed rather than my body. I could lift or lower my legs or my back or both and this helped a lot. Susan slept in the empty bed next to mine for my first night in the step-down unit.

I began to feel better. I was not in very much pain and only dosed myself with morphine once or twice. The step-down unit was my home for four days after the surgery. It was a large room with six beds. The nursing station was in the far corner, away from my bed. I was on multiple monitors and had several sacks of IV fluid attached to me through a special machine. I was attended by nurses who monitored and recorded many things. They took my temperature and blood pressure every four hours throughout the night. They recorded how much pain I had on a scale of one to ten. They noted the amount of urine I put out and the amount of saline that went in. They frequently took blood for tests. And they were right there if I needed them.

ACUTE CARE FLOWSHEET

Date: 24/08/05
Time: 7:30-12:00

CLINICAL NOTES

07:30 Patient having fainting episode. Dr. Choi and team at patient's bedside. Patient in trendelenburg position and remains conscious. Patient presently verbalizing with Medical Doctors (MDs). Normal Saline (NS) 1Litre (L) bolus started.

Signed: M. Johnson RN

07:45 Dr. Reznick and team in to see patient. Patient alert and oriented x 3. Blood Pressure (BP) 105/70. Rated pain 2/10. Patient Controlled Anesthesia (PCA) morphine remains on hold.

Signed: M. Johnson RN

08:15 Dr. Ashmalla in to assess patient. Patient's wife at bedside. No fainting episodes experienced.

Signed: M. Johnson RN

08:45 Patient complained of feeling sleepy and wanting to rest.

Signed: M. Johnson RN

09:00 Patient asleep but easily roused. Patient's wife at his bedside.

Signed: M. Johnson RN

09:30 Dr. Fenech in to assess patient. 1 unit Packed Red Blood Cells (PRBC) infusing. No untoward signs noted x 3. Family member at patient's bedside.

Signed: M. Johnson RN

AC FLOWSHEET CONTINUED	**Date: 24/08/05** **Time: 7:30-12:00**

10:00   BP 150/71. Patient oriented x 3. Abdomen soft. Urinary Output (U/O) adequate per hour. 1 unit of PRBC infusing.

Signed: M. Johnson RN

10:15   Outreach nurse was in to assess patient. Lasix 10mg Intravenous (IV) started as ordered. Patient reported having the urge to pass gas. Incentive spirometer used.

Signed: M. Johnson RN

10:33   Patient dozed off briefly. Lasix 10mg infused. 1L bolus infused continues while 2nd unit of blood is being requisitioned. Dr. S. Ashmalla in to see patient.

Signed: M. Johnson RN

11:00   1 unit PRBC started. Patient using incentive spirometer.

Signed: M. Johnson RN

12:00   Rated pain 2 / 10. Temperature (T) 37.4. Abdomen soft. No bleeding noted.

Signed: M. Johnson RN

APS CONSULT	**Date: 24/08/05** **Time: 11:20**

Acute Pain Service (APS) (McCluskey):
Post Operative Day (POD) #1, lap assisted right Hemicolectomy.
- Patient controlled anesthesia (PCA) morphine on hold since midnight due to fainting.
- Has not received any episodes since then.
- Continues to receive Toradol. Creatine = 90, Hemoglobin (Hb) = 84. Pain score 3/5.
- No nausea, no pruritus, no gas, no bowel movement (BM), nothing by mouth (NPO), patient being transfused.
Plan:
- Continue with Toradol as ordered.
- Resume PCA.
- Will reassess this plan.

Signature illegible

APS CONSULT	Date: 24/08/05 Time: 12:45

APS (McCluskey):
- Patient used 1.0 mg of his PCA with good relief.
- No fainting noted but felt like he was going to faint when he was dangling his legs.
- Pain score remains at 3/5.
- No nausea, no pruritus.

Plan: Continue with same treatment (Tx).

Signature Illegible

NURSING ASSESSMENT	Date: 24/08/05 Time: Day Shift

Name: Glouberman
MRN#: 2397544
Neurological/Psychosocial: - Patient drowsy but arousable. Patient had a brief fainting episode.
- Patient controlled analgesia (PCA) morphine on hold. Patient rated pain 2/10.
- Firm hand grip noted. Moving lower peripheries independent.
- Spoke in clear soft tones. Able to follow all verbal cuing well.
- Visited by wife and friend.
Respiratory: - Respiration (R) 20/min and effortless.
- Oxygen Saturation 100% on 4 L oxygen via normal pressure (N/P). Chest expansions symmetrical.
- Good air entry (A/E) noted. No shortness of breath (SOB), no cyanosis noted. Trachea in mid line.
Cardiovascular: - Blood pressure (BP) 155/77, heart rate (HR) 80 beats per minute (bpm). Patient on telemetry. Oxygen Saturation 100% on 4L oxygen via N/P.
- Right peripheral intravenous (PIV) with normal saline (NS) at 125cc/hr. NS 1L Bolus infusing at present. General skin color pink. Good skin turgor. Pedal pulses present and equal.
- Capillary refill < 2 seconds. No peripheral edema noted.
Gastro-Intestinal: - Patient remains nothing by mouth (NPO) x 5, puncture site of abdomen stained with old blood. Naval/umbilical area appeared reddish. Abdomen soft, bowel sounds (BS) absent. No distension noted. Patient reported having a bowel movement (BM) this a.m.
Genitourinary: - Foley catheter with urometer remains in situ and presently drained 55cc amber urine.

Signed: M. Thomson RN

Wednesday, August 24, 2005: Evening

The second night in the step-down unit became a hospital nightmare. The new nurse decreed that Susan had to find a place in the waiting room if she insisted on staying in the hospital. When she left, a new patient, who I will call "Mrs. Grant," was brought in and placed in the neighboring bed. I woke up to her arrival. She was talking to her daughter as she was being wheeled in. Her daughter stayed for a few minutes but said she would go home since her mother was okay. The daughter left and Mrs. Grant called for the nurse and told her that she was feeling thirsty and would like something to drink. The night nurse explained that after stomach surgery, patients were not allowed to take anything by mouth for several days. Mrs. Grant would have to wait until she was a bit better. "But I am thirsty," she insisted. It was now eleven o'clock at night. She began to shout for the nurse every few minutes, saying that she was very uncomfortable and insisting that she needed some juice. She became louder and more insistent as the night wore on. Just as I would drift off, she would shout, "Nurse! I'm thirsty!" The night nurse was sympathetic and commiserated with her and reassured her, but nothing helped.

NURSING ASSESSMENT	Date: 24/08/05 Time: Night Shift

Name: Glouberman
MRN#: 2397544
Neurological/Psychosocial: Patient asleep in bed. Easy to wake. Oriented x 3. Pleasant, co-operative. Verbalizes needs/concerns on patient controlled anesthesia (PCA) morphine. Stated 0/10 pain rate.
Respiratory: Pulse oximeter (Pox) – 20/min 022 liters normal pulse (NP) Saturation – 95%.
- Respiration regular, unlaboured, chest clear. Stated 1/5 for pain. No cough.
Cardiovascular: BP – 157/65, HR – 86 BPM, temperature (T) – 36.6. - Skin warm and dry to touch. Has no peripheral edema, peripheral pulse present (ppp) x 4 Rt. PIV in tact NS at 125cc/hr infused. Patient on tele-

NURSING ASSESSMENT CONT'D | **Date: 24/08/05**
Time: Night Shift

metry - normal sinus rhythm (NSR).
Gastro-Intestinal: Nothing by Mouth (NPO). Abdomen
soft, no distension, with no BS x 4. Abdominal wound
punctures x 5, no steri-strips, dry and intact (D&I).
Umbilical area pinkish.
Genitourinary: Foley in situ - draining amber urine.

Thursday, August 25, 2005

The nurse from the Critical Care Outreach Team came
to visit me in the stepdown unit. She woke me and was unin-
terested in the events of the night.

ACUTE CARE FLOWSHEET | **Date: 25/08/05**

CLINICAL NOTES

00:30   Blood transfusion completed. No blood reaction noted. Gravol 50mg intravenous (IV) given as
requested.

01:00   Asleep on and off. No complaints.

02:00   Asleep on and off. No complaints.

03:00   Asleep on and off.

04:00   Patient complained of not getting a good
night's sleep. Complaint of the hospital's management. Complained about noisy roommate. Complete
Blood Cell Count (CBC) RR sent.

05:00   Asleep.

CCOT CONSULT | **Date: 25/08/05**
Time: 05:15

Critical Care Outreach Team (CCOT) follow-up (F/U)
Day 2 Post Right Hemicolectomy. Originally paged
on day 1 post op for fainting spells. Patient has not
had issue with this for one day and blood pressure
remains stable. Issue currently = continual gradual

CCOT CONSULT CONTINUED	Date: 25/08/05 Time: 05:15

decline in hemoglobin (Hb) despite transfusions. Hb
@ 2000=87 1 unit packed red blood cells (PRBC)
given. 01:00 Hb=96 - 04:00 Hb=90.
Plan: Continue to monitor complete blood cell count
(CBC) for 3 hours please. Full blood work due @
07:00 - Registered Nurse (RN) agreeable. General
surgery resident aware and discussed possibility of
another operation (OR) with patient.

Thank you from CCOT, (416-790-9969)

Signed: A. Zakizewski RN

ACUTE CARE FLOWSHEET	Date: 25/08/05

CLINICAL NOTES

6:00   Resting. Asleep on and off.

7:00   CBC RR and blood sent.

Signature illegible

GENERAL SURGERY NOTES	Date: 25/08/05 Time: 07:20

Vital Signs Stable (VSS), afebrile, urinary output
(U/O) – 540cc, on 2 Litres (L) of oxygen via Nasal
Prongs (NP).

SUBJECTIVE (S): Patient complains of increase in
abdominal pain. No Nausea/Vomiting (N/V) (+) flatus.
No syncopal episodes overnight (O/N).

OBJECTIVE (O): Last hemoglobin (Hgb) = 90 at
04:24 (down from 96). Abdomen – soft, mild distension, mild tenderness in periumbilical area, (+) ecchymosis over incision.
Impression: Haemotology test results stable but Hgb
down.

Plan: 1) Frequent complete blood cell count (CBC), 2)
Consider Computerised Tomography (CT) scan

Signed: Brar Clinical Clerk 4 (CC4)

CCOT CONSULT

Date: 25/08/05
Time: 10:50

Critical Care Outreach Team (CCOT) Follow Up (F/U) 48 hr post consult. Received patient sitting in chair using oxygen 2 Litres (L) of oxygen via Nasal Prongs (NP). Oxygen Saturation 94%. Breathing easy. Appears comfortable.

OBJECTIVE (O):
Neurological (Neuro): Alert and oriented. Glasgow Comma Scale (GCS) 15. Patient complained of slight increase in abdominal pain left of mid incision as compared to yesterday. Abdomen soft. Passing flatus. Patient controlled anesthesia (PCA) morphine 10 mg used only.

Respiratory (R): 2 NP, Respiratory Rate (RR) 20, Oxygen Saturation 94-96%. Air entry (A/E) clear throughout. Using incentive spirometer. Productive cough, no expectorate.

Cardiovascular (CVS): On telemetry – report sinus Heart Rate (HR) 73, no ectopy. Blood Pressure (BP) 178/81. Afebrile. No overt bleeding. No calf swelling. Pulses x 4. Peripheral Intravenous (PIV) 1 unit normal saline (NS) @ 125/hr + 2935 cc/24hr. Urinary Output (U/O) 550cc/12hr. Complete Blood cell Count (CBC) done every 3 hours (g3h). Hemoglobin (Hbg) down 88 at 07:00 from 90 at 04:30.
Genitourinary: Foley 550cc/12hr. No issues.
Patient has had no fainting episodes today and felt well when transferred to chair. No dizziness, no headache, no nausea and vomiting.
Plan – will follow CBC, supplement magnesium sulfate (חחחחMgSO4).

CCOT pager # 790-9969
Signed: A. Zakizewski RN

APS CONSULT

Date: 25/08/05
Time: 11:20

Acute Pain Services (McCluskey)
Post Operative Day (POD) #2, Surgical Procedures (S/P) lap admitted right Hemicolectomy.
- Patient controlled anesthesia (PCA) given at 1.0mg.
- Pain score 0/4.
- No nausea, no pruritus, fainting episodes stopped.
- Nothing by mouth (NPO).
- Stating that he has not been able to sleep, requesting

APS CONSULT CONTINUED
Date: 25/08/05
Time: 11:20

something to help him sleep. Patient used to take
Valium 5 mg periodically to help him sleep.

Plan:
- Continue with same treatment.
- Ativan 0.5 mg Sublingual (SL) OP at bedtime (HS)
as needed (RPN)

Later that morning, Mrs Grant's daughter reappeared
and Mrs. Grant demanded that she bring her something to
drink. When no drink came, she yelled that her daughter
was of no help to her, had abandoned her, and was altogeth-
er useless. The daughter left. Mrs. Grant's doctor, a greying,
middle-aged man in a rather elegant white coat, dropped by
looking somewhat embarrassed. He told her she was on the
mend but should not drink. But to no avail. Her demands
evolved into a day-long litany. Mrs. Grant now began to say
that she wanted to go home. I watched as the day nurse became more and more upset by her demands and she began
to pepper her irritation with veiled, and then not so veiled,
threats of sedation. This drama intensified throughout the
day, and by nightfall, my increasingly active neighbour got
out of bed and began to say things like, "This is my house.
Get me something to drink or get out." "What are you doing here? I didn't ask you to come to my house. Get out."
She gradually became more insistent that she was in her own
house and that all the people in the unit were interlopers. The
day nurses seemed to have no way to deal with her except to
insist on the doctor's orders and to declare the "rules of the
ward." She was not calmed by this. In fact, their reactions to
her seemed to increase her anxiety and elicit ever more ex-
travagant responses. As the day wore on, they began to offer
her sedation, which she refused.

Misha sent the following e-mail:

Hello followers of surgery.

Today's news is all very good!

The fainting spells seem to have stopped completely. My father hasn't fainted since early yesterday (Wednesday) morning, his blood pressure is normal, and his hemoglobin is stable. The doctor thinks there may be a small bleed which may have contributed to the low hemoglobin and the fainting, but he's not sure, and if there is, the stable hemoglobin levels suggest it's taking care of itself.

My father was able to sit up in a chair today, a couple of times so far, and spent a half hour sitting up and reading the paper.

Best of all: Amid all our concerns about fainting and hemoglobin and blood pressure, my father's colon was quietly (and busily!) healing itself. The colon is working again, and my father will start eating again today, beginning with what the doctor described with the medical term "mush".

Everything seems to be completely on track now. I'll keep you posted with future updates, and will continue to pass on any messages to him.

- Misha

CCOT CONSULT **Date: 25/08/05**
Time: 15:10

Critical Care Outreach Team (CCOT) Follow-Up (F/U). Hemoglobin (Hgb) from 1100 up 91. No worsening of abdominal pain. Patient in no distress. Plan for full phosphorus oxide (PO4) decreased to 41. Consider supplement. Please call for any acute changes in patient's condition. Illegible.

Thank you CCOT 416-790-9969
Signed: A. Zakizewski RN

NURSING ASSESSMENT **Date: 25/08/05**
Time: Day Shift

Name: Glouberman
MRN#: 2397544
Neurological/Psychosocial: Patient complained of (c/o) feeling tired and sleepy. No c/o pain. Moving all peripheries well. Able to flex and extend limbs within natural limits. Pupils equal, react to light and accommodation (PERLA). Spoke in clear soft tones. Oriented x 3. Wife

NURSING ASSESSMENT CONT'D	**Date: 25/08/05** **Time: Day Shift**

Susan present.
Respiratory: Respiration (R) 20/min and effortless.
Non-productive dry coughs noted. Chest sounds clear
on auscultation with all lobes. Chest-expansions symmetrical. Trachea in mid line. No shortness of breath
(SOB) noted, no cyanosis noted.
Cardiovascular: Blood Pressure (BP) 178/81, Temperature (T) 39 degrees, Heart Rate (HR) 92 bpm and
regular. Right peripheral intravenous (PIV) normal saline (NS) at 125cc/hr. Good skin turgor. Skin warm and
dry. Capillary refill < 2 seconds. Pedal pulses present
and equal. No peripheral edema noted.
Gastro-Intestinal: Remains nothing by mouth (NPO).
Flatus passed. Abdomen soft and non-tender. No increased bleeding noted at puncture site with abdomen
slight reddish discoloration with umbilicus remains.
Genitourinary: Foley catheter and urometer remains in
situ and draining large amounts of clear yellow urine.

Signed: M Thomson RN

Thursday, August 25, 2005: Evening

By the time the night nurse reappeared, Mrs. Grant
was in a sorry state. Somewhat bedraggled but surprisingly
strong, she continued to call for the nurse and to vigorously
demand drink and tell everyone to leave. The night nurse
calmed her down. She took her on long walks and soothed
her anxiety by holding her hand and speaking quite softly. I
even had a bit of sleep.

I was awakened by more loud demands. Apparently the
night nurse had gone off for her meal break and Mrs. Grant
was not about to accept her substitute. Out of her bed and on
the march, she became angrier and more shrill, telling everyone to leave her home. The nurse told her that she had to take
something to calm her nerves. Security personnel came to the
unit and helped to sedate Mrs. Grant. She was removed to a
separate side room on the floor.

The night nurse reappeared, quite upset, and wondered
why they had to call in security and why Mrs. Grant had been

sedated. My third night in the hospital was full of this drama. I wondered at Mrs. Grant's physical strength, but also at the night nurse's capacity to calm her (more than at the other staff's inability to deal with her). Security staff were a new wrinkle in my hospital experience. I never saw Mrs. Grant again. After carefully examining the medical and nursing charts, my encounters with her are conspicuously absent. The only mention of Mrs. Grant in my chart is from the night nurse, who wrote that I did not get a good night's sleep and "c/o about noisy roommate at 4:00 AM on August 25."

My wife Susan is a psychoanalytic psychotherapist, and we often have discussions about the relation of psychoanalytic theory to practice. I have often argued that psychotherapy is a talent that can be sharpened by theory, but first one should make sure that people who enter the field have a propensity for making therapeutic interventions. Some people are more suited than others to understand and help people. The same holds for physical therapy: some physiotherapists have "good hands" and others do not. I believe that health care systems must winnow out those who have little talent for human engagement. I believe that there are people who by their very nature would further provoke Mrs. Grant and others who have an untrained ability to calm her. Training can and must help with this, but it may not be enough to overcome a lack of native ability. I think more and more that everyone who works in health care should have the ability to sympathize and be responsive to others as a prerequisite for their entry into the field.

NURSING ASSESSMENT	Date: 25/08/05 Time: Night Shift
Name: Glouberman MRN#: 2397544 Neurological/Psychosocial: Received patient on bed awake, alert, oriented x 3. Able to move all limbs. Good hand grips. PERLA. Respiratory: Breathing effortlessly, regular, chest clear	

NURSING ASSESSMENT CONT'D | **Date: 25/08/05**
Time: Night Shift

and good air entry noted, chest expansion symmetrical. No shortness of breath (SOB). No cyanosis.
Cardiovascular: Blood Pressure (BP) 174/72, Temperature (T) 36.8, Heart Rate (HR) 92 beast per minute (bpm).
Right Peripheral Intravenous (PIV) with Normal Saline (NS) at 125cc/hr. Skin warm and dry to touch, skin turgor good. Capillary refill satisfactory. Peripheral pulse present (ppp) x 3. No peripheral edema noted.
Gastro-Intestinal: Bowel Sounds (BS) present x 4.
Abdomen soft and mild abdominal distension noted.
Laparoscopic site and steri-strips intact and old blood stain noted.
Genitourinary: Foley catheter to urometer bag and sufficient amount of amber urine output.

Signature Illegible

Friday, August 26, 2005

GENERAL SURGERY NOTES | **Date: 26/08/05**
Time: 07:20

All Vital Signs Stable (AVSS), urine output (U/O) increased (+), no nausea and vomiting (N/V)

SUBJECTIVE (S): Patient doing well this a.m. (+) flatus. No nausea or vomiting, no appetite this a.m., no chest pain (CP), no shortness of breath (SOB), and no syncope. Ambulatory. Tolerated full fluid (FF).

OBJECTIVE (O): Hemoglobin (Hgb) = 97. Abdomen is soft, no distension, and non-tender.
Impression = Improving

Plan:
1) full fluids continued today
2) discontinue (d/c) foley
3) transfer to floor

Signed: Brar Clinical Clerk 4 (CC4)

Now I was once more alone at my end of the step-down unit. I was gradually improving, even though I had slept very little during the last few nights. I could sit up. I could lie down. Susan was there. The nurse reported that there were encouraging sounds coming from my stomach. On this morning, I had a small, very greenish-black bowel movement. My digestive tract was working again, and I could now eat soft foods. I was moved out of the step-down unit into my private room. The nurses from the step-down were congratulatory.

NURSING NOTES	Date: 26/08/05 Time: 08:00

Received Patient awake, alert and oriented x 3. Understands and obeys commands, verbalizes needs well. Patient controlled anesthesia (PCA) morphine there for patient's use. Pain rated 2-3/10. 0 mg used at this time. Respiration (R) = 20, unlabored breathing spontaneously as respiration assessment (R/A) oxygen saturation 94-95%. No shortness of breath (SOB), no cyanosis. Chest expansion equal and symmetrical bilaterally. Air entry (A/E) good, no adventitious sounds heard. Patient's skin dry and warm to touch. Capillary refill brisk. No ankle edema noted. Noted left peripheral intravenous (L PIV) 2/3 - 1/3 units 125cc. Bag changed to normal saline solution with 125cc. Blood pressure (BP) 165 / 70, pulse (P) 80, temperature (T) 37.3. BP appears high with no anti-hypertensives ordered. Foley with urometer in situ and patient draining adequate amounts of urine at this time.

Signed: John Cardella RN

NURSING NOTES	Date: 26/08/05 Time: 09:00

Foley discontinued (d/c) and patient tolerated well. Wife at bedside and patient tolerated full fluid tray well. No nausea or vomiting at this time. Patient encouraged to use incentive spirometer (I/S). Ambulated in the hall with highwalker. Accompanied by wife. Abdomen soft and slightly distended. 4 puncture sites sterile and stripped. Area is dry and intact (D+I). Bowel sounds (BS) heard, and flatulence. Patient remains on telemetry. Patient sitting in a chair reading.

Signed: John Cardella RN

I was recovering. I began to have other visitors, and I was encouraged to take short walks. When I got out of bed, it was necessary to disconnect me from the heart monitor and report this to the monitoring unit, lest they think that I had died and call another Code Blue. The morphine pump stayed with me.

APS CONSULT	Date: 26/08/05 Time: 11:50

Acute Pain Services (APS) McCluskey. Post Operative Day (POD) #3 S/P Lap oriented Rt. Hemicolectomy. PCA morphine at 1.0 mg. None used this a.m. Pain same = 0/2. No nausea, no fainting. Full Fluid (FF) Diet. Complained of insomnia even though he took Ativan 0.5 last night. Plan: Discontinue Patient Controlled Anesthetics (PCA). Ativan 1 mg (+) at bedtime (HS) as needed (PRN) under the tongue (SL).
Will sign off.

Signature Illegible

NURSING NOTES	Date: 26/08/05 Time: 12:30

Patient ambulated to next room on floor. Assisted back to bed. Family and friends visiting. Patient relaxing in bed reading a book. Vital signs stable (VSS). Patient enjoying lunch.

Signed: John Cardella RN

NURSING NOTES	Date: 26/08/05 Time: 15:00

Friends visiting. Patient sitting in chair and appears to be in good spirits. Telemetry still in use.

Signed: John Cardella RN

I continued to be closely monitored. I was told that Dr. Reznick would be away until the following Monday but his staff would take care of me and discharge me from the hospital when I was ready to leave. It was somewhat disconcerting that he was not around to help decide about letting me go home.

Hello.
  My father's recuperation is moving along speedily.
He's walking around the ward today. He's off the I.V.
and eating soup and ice cream.
  The doctors suspect there may have been a small
bleed after the surgery, but if there was, it has healed
completely.
  They hope to be able to send him home within a
couple of days. He'll then spend a few weeks at home
while his colon and abdomen continue to heal from
the surgery.
  I'm going out of town until Sunday. I'll send an update when I get back.
                                  - Misha

NURSING NOTES	Date: 26/08/05 Time: 17:00

Patient telemetry discontinued (d/c). Friends and family visiting. Up to and about (R) saline lock has been
flushed and is potent.

Signed: John Cardella RN

NURSING NOTES	Date: 26/08/05 Time: 18:00

Patient has denied having pain at this time. No
analgesic given today. Patient has refused analgesic
throughout shift. Patient ambulated in hall with son
this evening.

Signed: John Cardella RN

NURSING NOTES	Date: 26/08/05 Time: 21:00

Patient received 20:30 awake and alert 0x3. Up in
chair, visiting with family. Vital Signs (VS): Temperature (T) 37 degrees, Pulse (P) 73, Respiration (R) 20,
Blood pressure (BP) 170/62. Oxygen Saturation 96%
respiration assessment (R/A). Chest clear. Patient
reports cough. Encouraged to breathe deep and cough
while breathing. Abdomen soft, distended. Bowel
Sounds (BS) (+) x 4. Quadrants flatus (+) patient reports
bowel movement yesterday. No peripheral edema, peripheral pulses present (ppp). Patient reports itching

NURSING NOTES CONTINUED	Date: 26/08/05 Time: 21:00

on abdomen around puncture site. He believes it is hair regrowth and reports that it is tolerable. Puncture sites with steri-strips dry and intact. Patient reports no pain. No further concerns.

Signed: S.R. RN

NURSING NOTES	Date: 26/08/05 Time: 23:00

Patient requested sleep aid. Ativan 1 mg sublingual (SL) given.

Signed: S.R. RN

Saturday, August 27, 2005: Discharge

NURSING NOTES	Date: 27/08/05

00:30 Patient sleeping. Wife sleeping at bedside.
Signed: S.R. RN

03:00 Patient and wife asleep.
Signed: V. White RN

05:00 Asleep and wife at bedside.
Signed: V. White RN

06:00 Vital signs stable. Patient wanted to have shower.
Signed: V. White RN

07:00 Assisted patient with shower/shampoo. Ambulating well. Hoping to go home today.
Signed: V. White RN

GENERAL SURGERY NOTES	Date: 27/08/05 Time: 11:30

Afebrile, Vital Signs Stable (AVSS). Urinary Output (U/O) – 1400cc over 12 hours. Patient doing well overnight. Tolerating diet (DAT) well. No nausea, no vomiting (N/V), no chest pain (CP), no syncopal events, no flatus. Abdomen –soft, not tender, not distended.

GEN. SURGERY NOTES CONT'D   **Date: 27/08/05**
Time: 11:30

Plan: Discharge home today.
Received patient awake in bed. Wife in room. Vital
signs (VS) taken. Abdomen soft and slightly distended. 4 puncture sites dry and intact. Bowel sounds
(BS) heard. Patient had bowel movement this a.m.
Tolerating diet (DAT), no nausea or vomiting (N/V).
Patient hospital card and discharge summary sheet
with discharge instructions given. Patient eager to go
home. Hemoglobin (Hgb) 96. Dr. M. Hescoy notified,
patient okayed to go home. Prescriptions given.

Signed: John Cardella RN

My nurses in the regular ward responded more slowly than the ones in the step-down unit, but I needed very little help. I was walking and felt ready to go home. They provided me with a discharge summary, which I signed. I was eager to go home and begin to heal on my own. I left that afternoon, and I was assured that I could call the residents if anything was amiss. Our friends Jerry and Ruthy Portner also returned to Montreal; they had done their job. I would go home to recover in peace.

2391544
Glouberman, Seymour
6633950088 HA
41 Woodlawn Ave East
Toronto ON M4T 1B9

DISCHARGE SUMMARY

Diagnosis:
Procedure/Treatment: Lap Hemicolectomy

INFORMATION GIVEN TO PATIENT GUARDIAN

Activity: [ ] As Tolerated   [x] No Heavy Lifting
Diet: 6-8 weeks
                pt given d/c instruction sheet

MEDICATION
1. Tylenol #3 1-2 tabs q4   5.
2. Coloce 100mg PO 810   6.
3.   7.
4.   8.

Home Care [ ] Yes   [x] No f/u in 3-4 weeks

REHABILITATION FACILITY

Name: Telephone: (   )

FOLLOW UP APPOINTMENT WITH

[x] Doctor: Dr. Reznick   Telephone: (416) 340-4137
Date: Time:
[ ] Other: Telephone: (   )
Date: Time:

I hereby acknowledge receipt and understanding of the
instructions indicated above

Nurse's Signature   Patient/Guardian Signature
Signed: Dj Cude   Signed: S Glouberman

Discharge Date: 27 Aug 05   Time: 11:00
Method: Car
Destination: Home   Accompanied by: Wife

POST SURGICAL INSTRUCTIONS   **Date: 27/08/05**

Diet : You may not feel like eating for the first couple of
weeks after surgery. Eat small meals often (i.e., every
3-4 hours) for the first couple weeks after your surgery
so that you do not feel too full.

Exercise & Activity: Do not lift more than 10-20 pounds
for the first 6 weeks. Then, slowly increase to the
amount you normally lift. Walking is the only exercise
recommended in the first 6 weeks. Gradually increase
the distance and speed you walk. After 6 weeks,
gradually return to normal physical activities.

Driving: You should not drive while you are taking any
Tylenol # 2 or #3 or Percocet. You should not drive
while you are still in discomfort.

Sexual Activity: Sexual activity may be resumed when
you feel ready to do so.

Rest: It is normal to feel very tired in the first few weeks
after your surgery. You should nap when you feel tired.
Your sleep patterns will slowly return to normal after
the first few weeks.

Incision Care: If you have staples, arrangements will
be made to remove them. Small Steri-Strip tapes are
placed on the incision to provide some support. They
will fall off on their own and do not need to be removed.

INSTRUCTIONS CONTINUED   **Date: 27/08/05**

It is good to have a shower daily and to let the water flow over the incision. Do not soak in a bath until the wound is completely healed.

Call your surgeon if you see:
• Increased amounts of drainage
• Changes in the smell and appearance of the drainage
• New redness, swelling or new discomfort near the incision line
• Your incision coming apart

Pain Control: You will be given a prescription for pain medication when you go home. Most patients need this type of medication 2 to 3 times daily for the first one or two weeks after discharge. You may take one pill instead of two and at less frequent intervals as your pain decreases. You may take one or two plain Tylenol instead of the Percocet or Tylenol # 3 if you wish. Percocet and Tylenol # 3 can make you drowsy. They can also make you constipated. Drink a lot of fluid and eat fruit and vegetables to help with this. Call your doctor if you do not have a bowel movement in more than two days.

Call your surgeon if you still have pain after the first two weeks

Additional Cautions: Call your surgeon if you have:
• Persistent or increased abdominal pain, new types of pain after discharge
• Fever / Temperature greater than 38.2°C.

Contact Information: General Surgery Clinic at 416-340-4800 Ext. 8060 Monday to Friday between 07:30 am and 05:00 pm. If you require urgent attention after hours go to the nearest emergency department.

Our house has lots of stairs and our bedroom is on the second floor. I had worried about getting there on my own. I was assured that I could do it slowly without risk of hurting myself or pulling the stitches. I got home safely and I climbed the stairs to our bed. It was far more uncomfortable than the hospital bed – no way to adjust it for my pain. I had to sleep on my back because it was too painful to turn onto my side. Still, it was a pleasure to be home. My job was to blow into the little tube and make sure that I didn't get pneumonia.

Sunday, August 28, 2005

We monitored my temperature. I spent much of the day in bed, where I could not turn and was forced to sleep on my back. Every night, I woke up sweating and had to put on a new t-shirt at least once a night. I could sit up outside my bed and walk slowly up and down the stairs. Night sweats have since been a common occurrence. I walked with Susan every day, at first to the corner and back, and then just around the corner, at times with friends like Peter Moss, who was my weekly gym companion. My temperature stayed slightly above normal and I watched TV and read bad novels. I was feeling a bit better. I was home. Sunday was uneventful. I rested, read, and took my pills. I was recovering.

Chapter Three

Complications:
Second Hospital Stay

Monday, August 29, 2005

On Monday night, I got a high fever. Eileen was there delivering groceries, and she took us to the hospital to see what was happening. We entered the Emergency Department at seven p.m. and were immediately seen by Dr. Sahajpal and other residents who got us into a cubicle where blood was taken.

EMERGENCY SERVICES REPORT

Date: 29/08/05
Time: 17:04

DEMOGRAPHICS
Medical Record No.: 2397544
Visit No.: 252027908
Brought In By: Family Member
Referred to Physician/Telephone: Christopher Schneck/X3946

ALERT
Presenting Complaint: Fever (38.7)
Triage and Acuity Scale: Urgent
Time: 23:12

DISPOSITION
Consultation: General Surgery
Called: 19:10
Discharge Date: 30/08/05
Discharge Time: 01:15

CLINICAL NOTES
Give - to go as ordered by General Surgery.
Signature: Signature Illegible

MEDICATION
@ 01:10 Keflex 500mg by mouth (po).

Signature: Signature Illegible

CONSULTATION FORM   **Date: 29/08/05**

CONSULTATION FORM
DATE: August 29, 2005
REFERRING M.D.: Dr. Sahajpal
REASON FOR CONSULTATION: Direct to General
Surgery
CONSULTATION REQUESTED FROM: Emergency
Room
CONSULTANT'S SUMMARY:
ID: 65 year old man. Recent Laparoscopic Right-Hemi-
colectomy (Aug. 23) 6 days ago.
Reason for Referral (RFR/CC): Increase in tempera-
ture (39.2) at home – called Senior Resident – told to
come
Past Medical History (PMHx): 1) Laparoscopic Right-
Hemicolectomy for sessile villous polyp found on
screen C-scq
-       OR Aug. 23
-       Post Op bleed – hematoma RLQ/R-inguina; 3
units Packed Red Blood Cells (PRBC)
2)   HTN (recent)
Medications:
1)   Aspirin (ASA) 325 mg taken by mouth (po) OD
2)   Vitamins
3)   Salpalmeto
4)   Ginka Baloba
5)   Omega 3
6)   Glucosamine
Medical History (SxHx):
1)   Remote Tonsillectomy
Family History (FHx):
1)   Father/Uncle Colon Cancer
2)   IHD
3)   DM
Allergies: None Known (NKA)
HPI:
- August 27th discharged (D/C) from hospital
- Feeling well – noticed perspiration last night – T 38 at
18:00, no nausea, no vomiting, positive appetite, good
PO, ambulating – T 37.4 in the morning, no chills, no
rigors.
- 17:00 today T 39.2 – remains asymptomatic. No diarrhea, flatus, several BM, no BRBPR, no melena spots
post-op. No calf pain, no arm pain.
- No new pain around the incisions – diminishing – no
analgesics
- Hematoma – Sat, only noticed once he got home,
increase today
- Cough – yellow sputum, no hemoptysis, no H/A, no
neck pain, not stiff
- No dysuria, no urgency, nocturia – not new, no hematuria, no chest pain (CP), illegible – since OR

CONSULTATION FORM CONT'D   **Date: 29/08/05**

not truly Shortness of Breath (SOB) – no incentive spirometry.
– If there was no temperature and no perspiration, "would not know what was wrong"
On Examination: Looks well.
NAD: T = 38.6, BP = 145/72, P = 80, RR = 18, SpO2 = 97% RA.
HENT: Neck supple, reactive LA 6/1 greater than 1cm cervical nodes.
CVS: NHS, no S3, no S4, positive SEM III/VI over AO – no radiation JVP 4cm.
RESP: Decrease A/E on R base, mild crackles, no bronchial sounds.
ABDO: Bowl sounds (BS), large R-flank/LUQ/ R-hip hemotoma
LEGS: No peripheral edema, no tenderness of calves. soft/non-tender/non-distended, periumbilical erythema and warmth on scar, tense, not painful, no expression.
SKIN: Hematoma – R-flank, RLQ, R-hip, R inguina – confluent
DIAGNOSTICS:
98/87.8 – 11.9/9.8 - 233
(Aug. 29th Hb = 96)
Chest X-Ray (CxR): b/1 pleural effusions
URINE: pending
CT ABDO: pending – perianastomatic fluid (more likely hemotoma, no sign if free air or collection).
NB: Peri-umbilical erythema was marked before discharge, no significant increase.
Patient reviewed Post Operative Day (POD) #6 – febrile
– No respiratory SX
– No GI SX
– No coronary SX
– CT ABDO – no contrast reached anast minim/free
– Air – no collection – illegible units – hemotoma and air illegible
– O/E – illegible erythema, no drainage, non-tender
– Signature Illegible
Impression (IMP): fever likely 2 degrees to wound infected hematoma.
PLAN:
1)   Infected hematoma, open superior aspect of incision vs. conservative management
2)   Review CT with Radiology Staff
- Signed: CRZEH R
A/P: Patient stable, no obvious source. Will d/c with Keflex and reassess at clinic on Thursday morning. If any problems in interim to follow-up here. Discuss with Dr. Reznick.

Date: August 29, 2005
Consultant's Name: Dr. A. Sahajpal

They did an immediate X-Ray and decided to do a CT scan to see what my insides were like. A friend of ours, Alex Tarnopolsky, came to the hospital to stay with us, and Berl arrived shortly after.

I was given an hour to drink the contrast fluid – about a litre of white gunk that was reminiscent of the Colyte. Then they wheeled me out of the booth and into the CT scan room where a thin attendant told me that he had to introduce a further contrast fluid rectally. He inserted the tube and the fluid. He then put a needle into my arm and told me about the contrast medium that would be injected into my blood stream just as the CT scan was being done. It might make me feel warm; it could also cause other, more serious side effects like seizures, which they would monitor, and it could, in very rare cases, result in death. The CT scanner rumbled into action, and as the scan began, a taped, very British woman's voice told me when to hold my breath and when to breathe normally. The scan was over and the needle taken out. No side effects. I was returned to the booth and awaited Susan and Alex. Susan went off to get some coffee, and Alex and I were left alone in the cubicle to wait for the results of the scan. Soon, I began to feel as if I had to go to the bathroom – a bowel movement was imminent. As it became more and more urgent, I asked Alex to find out where the bathroom was or to get a bed pan for me. He left. Too late! I began to defecate uncontrollably. It was a sopping mess – all over the trolley, all over the floor, all over me. I was forewarned about everything but this. I had no seizure. I did not die. Instead, I was completely humiliated.

Alex returned, and when he saw me, he ran to get a nurse. She came back with an orderly while I remained in the shit and then shat some more.

"What was that about?" I asked. "No one told me that this might happen."

"They never tell us when they give you a contrast enema," the nurse said and proceeded to clean most of it up. They cleaned me completely, gave me a new gown, washed off the trolley and put me back on it. Traces of feces clung to the floor and shit was in the air.

I thought, "I did not consent to this."

What the CT scan attendant told me (and, of course, what he failed to tell me) was part of what is called "disclosure." The patient is told of the various possible side effects of a given procedure. The possibility that you might die is a rather uncomfortable preparation for having a CT scan. I later learned that this information is given to the patient not to help prepare them for the experience, but rather to avoid legal liability for untoward consequences. And so nothing is said about the feeling of confinement, the noise of the machine, or the possibility that the enema may result in a sudden incontinence.

The residents returned at about 12:30 a.m. with the results of the CT scan. There were several possible sources of infection, they said. There were several blood balls surrounding the connections where the resection had been done. It also looked like there might be some infection around the major incision in my navel. If I liked, they would cut open the incision then and there, clean it out, and let it heal. The other alternative was to increase the antibiotic and send me home hoping that the infection would clear up on its own. I decided to take the antibiotics because I did not want to have the wound opened unnecessarily. I was given several antibiotic pills that would work until we could get a prescription filled, and a follow-up appointment was made for Thursday morning in the Surgical Outpatients Clinic.

"The antibiotics should keep it under control until we see you on Thursday. You can go home now."

It was 1:30 a.m., Tuesday morning. Alex drove us home.

DEM NURSING ASSESSMENT	Date: 29/08/05 Time: 19:50

DEPARTMENT OF EMERGENCY MEDICINE NURSING ASSESSMENT
TGH/Urgent
Present Complaint: Fever
Triage Assessment: Today – cough, no increase in pain, given Tylenol x 2.
Related History: Bowel resection 1 week ago. Blood Pressure (BP) 168/79, Heart Rate (HR) 68, Respiration (R) 15, Temperature (T) 38.7.
Allergies: None Known
Medications: None
Last Tetanus Given: N/A
Method Of Arrival: Ambulatory
Assessment Obtained From Patient
Referral Letter: No

Initial Vital Signs: Left Arm: Supine: BP 145/70, Pulse (P) 80, Respiration Rate (RR) 18, T 38.6, Oxygen Saturation 97% RA

Triage Nurse's Signature: Signature Illegible
Primary Nurse's Signature: Signature Illegible
Initial Vital Signs: Left Arm: Supine: BP 145/70, Pulse (P) 80, Respiration Rate (RR) 18, T 38.6, Oxygen Saturation 97% RA
A)   Neurologic: Left Blank
B)   Cardiovascular: (i) Pulse – Regular; (ii) Skin – No abnormalities, warm; (iii) Chest Pain – N/A
C)   Respiratory: (i) Rhythm – Regular; (ii) Depth – Adequate; (iii) Quality – Adequate; Air Entry – A/E Bilaterally
D)   Abdominal: Left Blank
E)   Genitourinary: Left Blank
F)   Musculoskeletal: N/A
G)   Spine & Pelvis: N/A

Nurse's Signature: Illegible

NURSING NOTES	Date: 29/08/05 Time: 19:55-01:15

19:55 Presents to Emergency Room (ER) complaining of fever. The same started at about illegible today. History of bowel resection 1 week ago. Seen by General Surgery. Blood drawn and sent. Illegible. Illegible

21:00 General Surgery still seeing patient. Illegible

22:00 Taken to Ct. Illegible

NURSING NOTES CONTINUED   **Date: 29/08/05**
                            Time: 19:55-01:15

23:00 Returned from CT. Incontinent and says small amounts of stool. Linens and gown changed. Illegible

00:30 General Surgery still assessing patient. Illegible

01:10 Medication given as prescribed. Illegible

01:15 Patient discharged with prescription for Keflex 500mg by mouth (po). Illegible

Discharged at 01:15 accompanied by wife.

Means of discharge: Ambulatory

CT ABDOMEN REPORT   **Date: 29/08/05**
                           Time: 22:30

Location   Name
DIS EP   Glouberman, Seymour
MRN #   Visit #   Sex   Age
2397544   252027908 M   65Y
Abdomen Computed Tomogram
Tue, 30 Aug 05 1030 Documented by
Accession**: 301729911
Read By: Martin E. O'Malley, MD
Date Dictated: 30Aug2005
Exam Report:
REPORT (VERIFIED 2005/08/30)

CT ABDOMEN: Axial volumetric acquisition from the levels of the hemidiaphragm to ischial tuberosity done with IV and oral contrast.
Small bilateral pleural effusions right more than the left with basal atelectasis noted.
Within the abdomen, the liver demonstrates multiple low density lesions with the largest measuring approximately 1.2 x 0.8 cm in segment 4A. These are most likely to be cysts.
Normal adrenals, pancreas, spleen. The left kidney demonstrates a non-obstructing stone at its mid pole measuring approximately 0.8 cm.
There is a small focal collection measuring 2.8 x 3.4 cm adjacent to the right kidney in the anterior pararenal space associated with thickening with of the Gerota fascia. Further small pocket of fluid is seen in the left paracolic gutter. There is some high density material seen around the anastomosis site with a Hounsfield unit of approximately 50 which would be consistent with small hematoma at this site.

75

CT ABDOMEN REPORT CONT'D   **Date: 29/08/05**
                            Time: 22:30

I do not see any extraluminal contrast nor free gas within the abdomen to suggest anastomotic leak. No large focal collection or abscess is noted in this study. Bones demonstrate no significant pathology. Minimal soft tissue stranding is noted around the incision site consistent with post surgical change.

CONCLUSION: No evidence of anastomotic leak or large collection is seen in this study. Soft tissue high density material seen around the anastomosis is most likely to represent post-operative hematoma.
ECl/ap

Tuesday, August 30, 2005

We went home and I slept a bit. In the morning, I felt better. The fever went down. The antibiotics were working. They would last until Friday. The infection did not hurt in the area of the big incision, which was still taped. I was okay. I would be okay.

All day Tuesday, I napped and read and watched television. Misha and Margaux came for dinner. I was pretty tired and remained quite upset about the evening before. It felt like a bit of a nightmare. But it had passed. It would be okay now. We even celebrated a bit.

That evening, I was adjusting the blanket, making myself more comfortable in bed. I looked down and saw what appeared to be a pink fluid oozing out of the bandage over the main incision. In fact, there was quite a lot of it. The sheet was wet. My underclothes were wet. Susan called the resident.

Dr. Reznick was on holiday for the week. Dr. Choi, the resident on call, said that I needn't come in for the second night in a row; she would see me the following morning. The good news was that we now knew where the infection was and we could clean it up. Now that it was leaking, we would have to cut it open and clean it out. It would not clear by itself.

Wednesday, August 31, 2005

A somewhat restless night was followed by a trip to the hospital by cab the next morning. Dr. Choi was waiting for us in the outpatient area. She had a more junior person with her – a trainee surgeon. She injected a local anesthetic and asked me if it was okay for him to cut the sutures. He groped the tweezers and scissors, searching for the sutures, finding them and taking them out. She herself then quickly and without any fuss opened the wound and cleaned it. "This will leave you with a bit of an ugly scar, but it should heal in a week or two."

"What about the antibiotics?" I asked.

"Take them until they run out. You'll be fine."

The outpatient nurse then packed the wound, put a bandage over the opening, and explained that the wound could not be stitched up again. It had to heal from the inside out and would have to be cleaned and repacked every day until it closed over and was completely healed. She said that she would be available to us as long as we needed her; we needed only to call. She herself might call us to see how it was going. She then gave us over to the Home Care Coordinator, who would arrange for a nurse to come to the house to do wound care. The coordinator met us and gave us a bag of materials that included bandages, saline solution, tweezers, and packing material so that the home care nurse could come the next day. She also gave us a set of instructions about how to sterilize the necessary bits.

CHART COPY

Date: 31/08/05

NAME: Glouberman, Seymour
DOB: 10 October 1940
MRN: 239 7544 G
VISIT #: 251010054
LOCATION: Active IP
Date Dictated: 31Aug2005

CHART COPY CONTINUED   **Date: 31/08/05**

Date of Visit: 31Aug2005
Mr. Glouberman was seen today in clinic with regards
to his midline incision at the periumbilical site. It appears that he has had purulent drainage from this and
no resolution of the erythema, despite p.o. antibiotics. We thus opened this and packed this incision
today with saline soaked gauze. There was actually a
minimal amount of pus from the wound, however, due
to the significant cellulitis surrounding it, we felt that this
was the proper thing to do. He was sent home with
Home Care and a follow-up appointment as previously
arranged.
Thank you.
Dictated by: Dr. J. Choi
Service of: Richard K. Reznick, MD, Med, FRCSC,
Professor of Surgery, University of Toronto
Department of Surgical Oncology
Tel: 416-34-4137 | Fax: 416-595-9846
E-mail: richard.reznick@utoronto.ca
cc. Dr. Robert Kingstone, MD
Dr. To Patient Unknown, MD
Dr. Richard K. Reznick, MD

We were home by 11:00 a.m., and now that the infection
was gone, I was pretty tired and somewhat weak, so I rested
for all of Wednesday.

Thursday, September 1, 2005

The next morning we got a call from home care: a nurse
would come. Sonia was an articulate, lively woman who
said that she would start me off. She would not be my nurse:
someone else called Rachelle would come to take care of me.
She looked at the wound and said, "Ooh this is pretty deep
– it will take a good six weeks to heal, maybe eight."

My heart dropped. I was looking forward to swimming
in two weeks and going back to work by then. I could wait a
bit longer, but six weeks as a semi-invalid did not feel good.
"Can I swim?" I asked.

"I don't think so," she said. "You don't want to get chlo-
rine in an open wound and you don't want to bathe either.

You can shower in the morning before the nurse arrives and then she can dry and clean the wound. I will order materials for Rachelle that should get here by this afternoon. Here are some instructions for caring for the wound."

What a difference this made to me at the time. I would have to defer swimming for such a long while. When would I be able to go back to work? What did the resident think to say this was a two week wait? How far off she was. Was it ignorance? Was it excessive optimism? Was it the desire to avoid giving me bad news? Was it an attempt to mitigate the damage that had already been done?

SPECTRUM HEALTH CARE
A Commitment to Excellence

Instructions For Clients Who Require Dressings:

Your Doctor has ordered treatment which includes a dressing change. In order to carry out the dressing change, your nurse needs you to gather the following equipment and to prepare it according to the directions outlined below. The nurse will review this with you during your visit.

Please gather the following equipment:

-- Medium or large size pot with tight fitting lid
-- Microwaveable container with lid (if using microwave)
-- A small boilable glass dish (E.g. Pyrex or baby food jar)
-- Plastic bag (E.g. grocery bag) for dirty dressings
-- Towel (to protect your furniture)
-- Paper Towel
* The nurse may add to this list

Preparation of the Equipment:

A. Put glass dish and other supplies as needed into the pot / microwave container
B. Fill pot / microwave container with sufficient tap water to cover supplies
C. Bring pot / container to a rolling boil
D. Continue boiling for ten minutes (10)
E. Turn off heat - DO NOT REMOVE LID
F. Leave pot at room temperature to cool
G. The nurse will remove the lid when he/she gets there

** Please prepare the equipment well in advance of the visit so that there is time for the equipment to cool down.

Forms\Nsg. Chart\Dressing Instructions for clients/June, 1997 Rev. March, 2003

My Operation

Friday, September 2, 2005

On Friday morning, Rachelle herself arrived. She drove up in her car – the license reading "CNTRYGRL." Rachelle had long blond hair and was indeed a country girl. She was friendly and forthcoming.

"Hi. I'll be takin' care of yer wound till it gets better. Let's take a look at it. Are the supplahs here? Oohh, that's a deep wound. It'll take about six'r seven weeks to heal...But someone'll be here every day, seven days a week, to repack the dressing, and it'll get better."

She looked at the supplies, which had arrived the day before. "They sent a whole lot of stuff that ah don't like. Wooden sticks are no good. Ah need plastic ones. The ribbon for packing is much better in little sections than in bottles. But don'tcha worry, ah have stuff in the car." And she went out to the car and brought in more supplies. She talked about her work quite a lot. She delighted in telling us about her long day that began at 6:00 a.m. and could include between ten and fourteen patients.

Saturday, September 3, 2005

Saturday night came only too quickly. It was my cousin Linda's daughter's Bat Mitzvah. I thought that I might be able to go, but in the event, I could not. Susan went. All my cousins had come to Malka's Bat Mitzvah with their kids. They all were concerned about me and asked after me. My brother Nochom stayed with us. He and his wife Dena had to stay in the basement because I was using the guest room to read and rest. My fever remained low grade through the weekend.

Sunday, September 4, 2005

I felt well enough to go to a family party on Sunday. Nochom drove us there. He was planning to stay at the party

80

for a little while. He would then drive us home and continue to Montreal, where he lives. This suited me because I was not sure how long I could last before I got tired. I stayed for about a half hour and began to feel very tired and somewhat ill. I said goodbye, went out to the car, and sat down on the hood waiting what seemed like forever for my brother to finish his goodbyes and take me home. We went home. My fever went up and I felt a bit sicker, but nothing unusual. A long night and I became sicker. Our friends Steve and Marcia came to visit, but I was pretty much out of it. Perhaps I had done too much. Going out was still beyond my capacity.

Monday September 5, 2005

I woke up on Monday morning shivering and shaking. I could hardly move. Susan ran to George and Wendy, our neighbours, and told them that I had become very ill and needed to be taken to the hospital. George came immediately and helped me get dressed; I could hardly put on my trousers by myself. I needed help buttoning my shirt and putting on my shoes. Two winter coats covered my shivering, and George helped me into his car. We arrived at the emergency room to a waiting resident. I was freezing.

NURSING NOTES

**Date: 05/09/05
Time: 12:40**

Admitted to unit at 11:30 a.m. from emergency accompanied by wife. Patient alert and oriented. Intravenous (IV) normal saline (NS) in progress. Tentative diagnosis: Abdominal abscess. Vital signs stable (VSS): Temperature (T) 37 degrees. Abdominal dressing intact. Dressing done in emergency and antibiotics given in emergency. But large purpuric area on right side. Dr. Khumar aware. Settled in bed. Assessment taken. Wife at bedside.

Signed: V. White RN

IR REPORT

Date: 05/09/05
Time: 13:31

INTERVENTIONAL RADIOLOGY

Chart Review Print
Name: Glouberman, Seymour
MRN #   Visit #   Sex   Age
2397544 251013277 M   65Y
Physician Reznick, Rich
Status: complete
Percutaneous Drainage of Abscess - Abdomen
Event Time: Tue, 06 Sep 05 0849 Documented by
Accession*: 301736158
Read By: Martin E. Simons, MD
Date Dictated: 05Sep2005
Exam Report:

REPORT (VERIFIED 2005/09/06)

CT GUIDED ABSCESS DRAINAGE

INDICATION: The patient had a right hemicolectomy
performed 6 days back. On CT scan, there is a collection near the site of the anastomosis.

PROCEDURE: Informed consent was obtained.
The site of skin entry was planned on CT scan.
This site was cleaned and prepped and 10 cc of
local anesthetic was infiltrated all the way up to the
collection. 10 French multipurpose Dawson-Mueller
drain was inserted into the collection. About 40 cc of
reddish-brown fluid was aspirated. The drain was
connected to a bag. The patient tolerated the procedure well. 50 meg of Fentanyl and 1 mg Versed
were given during the procedure.

CONCLUSION: 10 French drain inserted under CT
guidance with satisfactory drain position.

DOCTOR'S ORDER SHEET

Date: 05/09/05

Physician's Signature: A. Sahajpal, Z. Yasser

Accurate input and output (I+O). Admit to Dr.
Reznick. Heparin 5000 units sc. twice a day (bid),
Zantac 150 mg po bid, can have antibiotics, can
have intravenous (IV) as ordered. Complete Blood
Cell Count (CBC), lytes, illegible in the morning
(a.m.). Continue pending changes.

Although I didn't know it, I had symptoms of septi-cemia. The system kicked in; the reaction was immediate. Acute hospitals are especially well able to deal with such episodes. And it is even possible that the rapid and effective response saved my life. Death from septicemia is hardly un-known, and if it had remained untreated, I would certainly have died. The medical attachment to acute conditions is oddly similar to the culture of public safety systems. Like doctors and nurses, police and firemen are at their best when responding to acute situations. In fact they prefer them to the boring activities associated with crime and fire prevention. My friend Lionel Stapeley told me that when he was a police-man at Scotland Yard, no one enjoyed the job of "keeping the grass free of dog shit."

They quickly began a series of tests. I was sent for an X-Ray. I was then sent for a new CT scan. Berl and Eileen came quickly to be with Susan.

"I'm sorry, but only one person can accompany the pa-tient," said the nurse.

"Berl will come with me," replied Susan firmly.

CONSULTATION FORM   **Date: 05/09/05**

CONSULTATION REQUESTED FROM:
General Surgery

REASON FOR CONSULTATION:
September 5, 2005 Post-Op Fever

CONSULTANT'S SUMMARY:
Mr. Glouberman is a 64 year old man who had a lap-aroscopic right hemicolectomy August 23rd, 2005 for villous polyp by Dr. Reznick. He went home August 27th, 2005. He came back to the Emergency Room on August 29th for wound infection. The wound was open and patient was given Keflex for 7 days. He just finished yesterday. The home care nurse was pack-ing the wound. A CT Scan on August 29th showed no leak but there was hematoma around anastomosis. The patient came in with rigors, a temperature of 39 degrees, but no pain. No meal last night tolerated well.

CONSULTATION FORM CONT'D   **Date: 05/09/05**

On Examination: Temperature 39, Heart Rate 130, Blood Pressure 150/75 The wound is clean and healing well. There is some redness around the wound. Soft abdomen, no peritonitis.

Plan: Intravenous (IV) fluid, blood works, swabs and cultures, IV antibiotics, CT scan abdomen, R/O intra-abdominal abscess VS leak.

Signed: Dr. Z. Yasser

DOCTOR'S ORDER SHEET   **Date: 05/09/05**

Tylenol 315-650mg po every 4hours as needed (PRN). Gravol 25-50 po/IV every 4 hours PRN. After cultures drawn: Maxiflaxacin 400mg IV every 24 hours; Flagyl 500mg IV every 12 hours; Amprillin 1g IV 6 hours. Computerized Tomography (CT) abdomen/pelvis.
Pack ribbon gauze wet with NS once per day.

The scan showed that the blood ball had grown and that it might be the cause of the septicemia.

I was then sent to the interventional radiology unit where they would try to suck out the big blood ball.

IR ORDER   **Date: 05/09/05**
        Time: 14:35

Interventional Radiology Orders:
NO Dr. Taneja/ illegible

1)   Fentanyl 50mg IV
2)   Midazolam (Versed) 1mg IV
3)   3 Litres of oxygen via nasal prongs
4)   C+S of aspirate by mouth

1 of Multipurpose drain inserted. Connected to bag. Sample obtained, sent for analysis.

Signature Illegible.

I was wheeled into a room about the size of a large class-room. It was painted white and had a windowed observation suite at one end. It was full of equipment – large scanners, ul-trasound machines, X-Ray equipment, and other machines that I could not recognize. The four people in the room were dressed in white and all smiles. I had entered their sanctuary, and they were happy to have me there. Cheerful and grinning, "Hello, I'm Dr. Simons and this is my colleague and here are our assistants," pointing to the pretty women who were not smiling and looked very business-like. "And we're going to fix you right up. We have everything we need right in this room."

"Just look at it," I thought, amazed at the amount of stuff. It was high-tech heaven.

"And you won't feel a thing; we're going to make you very happy first and then get down to business. What is your busi-ness by the way?"

"I do health policy research," I said tentatively, hoping to give the impression that I was somehow in the same business.

"So what do you think about private health care?" he said challengingly.

"I think it's quite a bad idea because it would result in two tier medicine," I said.

"We like the idea of two tiers," he said. "It would take the pressure off the rest of the system. But you have nothing to worry about; we'll still take care of you now and fix you right up."

"Let's see. I think we'll try to get that blood ball using the ultrasound machine first. If that doesn't work we'll go to the CT scanner."

They wheeled me up to the ultrasound.

"We'll find that blood ball and then we'll insert a tube to just suck it out. That will take out all the infected blood."

"Can you see where we have to go?"

"Nah. I think we need the CT."

So they wheeled me over to the CT scanner and tried again.

85

"There it is. I think we've got it all. Another scan and we can see. Yup. We got it."

"Now we're going to leave the tube in so it can drain. How do you feel?"

I thought that I felt like Lord Ashley, who later became the Earl of Shaftesbury. He was John Locke's patron and an early beneficiary of a tube that drained infection from his body. In 1668, after Ashley had terrible pains in his swollen abdomen, Locke, with the help of Thomas Sydenham, decided to treat him by opening his side to let it drain and then later inserting a silver tube to keep the passage open. Ashley kept the tube for the rest of his life, cleaning it with wine. He was forever grateful to Locke for relieving his pain. This was widely known at the time, and the press began to refer to Ashley as "Tapski." Sir William Osler later described the case in some detail as a significant event in John Locke's medical career.

Would I be forever grateful to the superheroes of interventional radiology?

I now had a tube too. It issued into a little plastic bag that was attached to my side. It had a little valve that allowed it to be emptied.

I was wheeled back to my room. I was once more the complete hospital patient with tubes going in and tubes coming out. I was monitored for blood pressure, and the intravenous drip included saline solution and antibiotic. My stomach had shut down again from the septicemia, so the nurses came to listen again for any sound of motion. There were more tests.

NURSING NOTES	Date: 05/09/05 Time: 16:00-18:15

Time: 16:00
Patient returned from interventional radiology at 15:05. T 37.2 degrees, Blood Pressure (BP) 130/80, Oxygen Saturation 98%. Right multipurpose drain in situ, dark blood drainage in tube only. Patient reassessed (R/A) by Dr. Khumar as he complained of pain

NURSING NOTES CONTINUED	Date: 05/09/05 Time: 16:00-18:15

in right hand before going down to interventional (no pain now). IV infusion via pump. Ice chips for mouth comfort and also swabs. Patient to remain nothing by mouth (NPO). Lots of family at bedside.
Signed: V. White RN

Time: 18:00
Meals given. Patient would like to eat. Dr. Khumar explained to patient and family on his return from interventional radiology that she would like him to remain on NPO. Dr. Khumar will speak to him again.
Signed: V. White RN

Time: 18:15
Received patient in bed. Aware, alert, oriented x 3. Vital signs stable (VSS). Air entry (A/E) clean bilaterally. No chest pain (CP), no adventious sounds noted. Abdomen slightly distended, soft bowel sounds (BS) present: No flatus noted as stated by the patient that he did not pass any flatus today as well. No bowel movement (BM). Abdominal dressing with slight serosang discharge (d/c). Right drain to straight drainage (SD) bag with dark red d/c. Small amount. Patient reports urinating independently. No edema noted to the feet. Peripheral pulse present (ppp) bilaterally, Homan's sign is negative bilaterally. Left ventricular intravenous (LPIV) infusing normal saline (N/S) @ 125cc/hr. Patient rates pain as 1.5/10 at this time.

Sent: Monday, September 05, 2005 8:12 PM
To: Friends Family And Colleagues of Sholom Glouberman
Subject: Latest update.

Hi,

I wanted to update a few of you on the state of my father's condition. While his colon seems to be healing well since he returned home from the hospital last weekend, the past week has been quite exhausting, with a series of continued symptoms, complications, discomforts and worries, marked by fevers, pains, and infection at the incision.

Sept 5 2005

My father was re-admitted to the hospital today, after ongoing fever and related symptoms. It appears that there was an abscess near the site of the surgery, which is likely to have been the cause of the fever and related problems.

> The doctors located the infection with a CT scan and drained it in the afternoon. My father's staying in the hospital for a night or two as they monitor his condition. My mother is staying with him.
>
> I gather that it's not uncommon to have this type of infection after surgery on the colon, and that while the immediate consequences have been unpleasant, the infection does not suggest any serious risk. My father wanted me to let work colleagues know that while he'd expected to be able to participate in calls and emails in the next couple of days, this will not be possible.
>
> - Misha

NURSING NOTES   **Date: 05/09/05**
                                 Time: 21:30-23:50

Time: 21:30
Patient is awake. Resting in bed and no voiced complaints at this time.

Time: 22:30
Ativan 1mg by mouth (po) given as needed.

Time: 23:50
Vital signs stable (VSS). Asleep but easily awoken. Signature Illegible

For Monday night, Susan had slept on a gurney cart next to me. But after that, she put a mat on the floor by my bed and slept there every night of my stay in the hospital. She found that she could not stay away; she could go off for coffee and take meals in the cafeteria, but it was too hard for her to be away overnight. On this second time around, I found her loving presence comforting and an enormous help. No one seemed to mind. If they did, no one said anything about it. Every morning, Susan and I nervously awaited the arrival of the residents. She now slept on the far side of my bed and would get up at 6:30 to make herself presentable for their arrival.

Tuesday, September 6, 2005

<table>
<tr><td>NURSING NOTES</td><td>**Date: 06/09/05**
Time: 01:00-06:15</td></tr>
</table>

Time: 01:00
Asleep on rounds.

Time: 02:00
Asleep on rounds.

Time: 03:00
Asleep but easily awoken. VSS.

Time: 05:30
Patient is awake. Resting in bed.

Time: 06:15
Patient is awake. Urinated 300cc of urine. No voiced complaint of discomfort at this time. Continue to monitor.

<table>
<tr><td>GENERAL SURGERY</td><td>**Date: 06/09/05**</td></tr>
</table>

Afebrile, Vital Signs Stable (AVSS); Temperature (T) 37.2 degrees.
Urinary Output (U/O) 600cc/shift. Pancreatic drain10 cc/shift.
Patient doing well. Slept well. Complained of pain on and off. Patient improving with no fever.
Clear Fluids (CF) – Diet as tolerated (DAT) today after discharge (D/C).
Signed: Dr. Reznick, Dr. Zaid Yasser

<table>
<tr><td>NURSING NOTES</td><td>**Date: 06/09/05**
Time: 11:00-20:00</td></tr>
</table>

Time: 11:00
Received patient resting in bed at 08:00. T. 37 degrees. Peripheral intravenous (PIV) normal saline (NS) at 125cc/hr via pump. Right drain draining very small amount of heavily bloody fluid. Bowel sounds (BS) and chest clear. Large bruised area on right side. Abdominal incision dressings packed with 1/4 inch gauze (wound looks clean). Wound swab taken and sent. Patient had a large semi-solid bowel move-ment (BM) at 10:00. Assisted patient with washing up.

Reassured and made comfortable. Meds given. Is now on sips of clear fluids.
Signed: V. White RN

Time: 12:00
T 37 degrees, IV in progress, antibiotic hung. Drain draining small amounts of bloody fluid. Abdomen large and soft. Dressing in tact. Wife at bedside.
Signed: V. White RN

Time: 15:00
T 37 degrees. Tolerating sips of clear fluid. States that he feels tired. Wife at bedside.
Signed: V. White RN

Time: 17:15-18:00
Temperature (T) 38 degrees, intravenous (IV) infusing. Patient's wife anxious. Complete blood cell count (CBC) drawn and seen by MD. Can now have clear fluids (CF) – diet as tolerated (DAT). Tylenol 2 given. Antibiotics in progress. DAT tray given as patient tolerated sips of clear fluid. Wife at bedside.
Signed: V. White RN

Time: 20:00
Received patient in bed. Awake, alert, oriented x 3. Vital signs stable (VSS). Air entry (A/E) clear bilaterally. Patient rates pain 3.5/10. Left peripheral intravenous (PIV) infusing normal saline (N/S) @ 125cc/hr. Abdomen slightly distended, bowel sounds (BS) present. Increase (+) in flatus and one bowel movement (BM) today. Abdomen dressing dry and intact (D&I). Right drain – straight drainage (SD) with very scant amount of dark bloody discharge (d/c). Patient reports urinating independently. No edema to the feet.

Physician's Signature: Signed: Dr. Yasser, V. White, RN Sips of clear fluid to diet as tolerated (DAT). Checked at 19:50 hours. Ativan 1mg po ghs x 1 dose. Transfer over from Dr. A. Abujazia to Merino

Signature Illegible

Wednesday, September 7, 2005

NURSING NOTES

Date: 07/09/05
Time: 01:00-08:00

Time: 01:00
Patient urinated 220cc of concentrated urine.

Time: 02:00
Asleep on rounds.

Time: 03:15
T 38 degrees. Tylenol extra strength (ES) 2 tabs po given.

Time: 05:30
Patient is asleep at this time.

Time: 06:15
Patient is resting in bed. No voiced complaints at this time. Seems comfortable. Continue to monitor.

Time: 07:15-08:40
Received patient lying in bed. Awake, alert and oriented x 2. Vital signs stable (VSS), afebrile. Left Peripheral Intravenous (PIV) site clean with normal saline (NS) @ 125cc/hr infusing well. Chest clear, no shortness of breath (SOB), no chest pain (CP). Abdomen soft and non-tender. Abdominal dressing changed and old dressing has small amount of new purulent drainage. Cleaned with NS and packed with 1/2 4 saline soaked ribbon gauze, covered with 4x4 medipore tape. Patient tolerated procedure well. No edema. Bowel sounds x 4 present, positive flatus and bowel movement. Pain minimal at this time. Wife at bedside. Patient going for abdominal x-ray (AxR) this morning. Will monitor. Call bell within reach.

ID CONSULT

Date: 07/09/05

Infectious Diseases (ID) Staff: Seems to be improving. Abscess/Right Lower Quadrant (RLQ) Collection decreased. Afebrile. Suggest: Continue same intravenous (IV) prescription (Rx) for another 2-3 days. Then step down to Clavulin if can take by mouth (po) Rx.

| DOCTOR'S ORDER SHEET | Date: 07/09/05 Time: 07:30 |

Physician's Signature and Order: Dr. Z. Yasser. T/O Dr. Huseynova to C. Arcarn, Start abdomen X-Ray. Infectious Diseases Consult on Chart. CT for today entered in PC.

| CF REPORT | Date: 07/09/05 Time: 12:00 |

COLORECTAL FELLOW (CF) REPORT
ID: 65 year old man now Post Operative Day (POD) #16 for laparoscopic assisted right hemiocolectomy for villous adenoma.
Course Post Op: History from patient.
POD # 1: Syncopal from retroperitoneal bleed (unknown at the time, patient presented with bruising later). Over 3.5 L crystalloid + 2 units packed red blood cells (PRBC). Was dynamically stable with soft abdomen in the a.m.
POD # 4: Sent home Aug. 27
POD # 6: Sudden on site rise in fever and chills. Patient states he had a small amount of abdominal pain, but had been eating well. Into Emergency Room (ER) – CT Scan collection around anast – not drainable. Sent home on antibiotics (Abx).
POD # 13: (Sept.5) Back to ER with vigors and Temperature (T) 39 degrees. Blood cultures drawn. Some upper abdominal discomfort. Fluid collection drained. Blood cultures positive for bacilli. Also, wound infection drained.
Functional Inquiry: Increase (+) in cough – sputum yellow with no dysuria. Bowel movement (BM) daily – none today.
Currently: bloated, slightly nauseated, no BM today, no gas today yet, no abdominal pain, no dysuria, no green, (+) yellow sputum.
On Examination (O/E): Temperature (T) 38 degrees max, vital signs stable (VSS).
Abdomen soft. Wound infection slightly bloated. X-ray done today.
Investigation: CT scan – small collection around anastomosis Sept.3.
Labs: (+) blood culture given – Sept. 3. White blood cell count (WBC) 11 up from 8-9, 2 days ago.
Impression: This gentleman has had 3 post op problems: #1 Retropentoneal heratona Post Operative Day (POD) #1 – now resolving. #2 Intra abdominal abscess – either due to chance contamination or minor anastomotic leak. #3 Wound infection.

CF REPORT CONTINUED

Date: 07/09/05
Time: 12:00

Diagnosis (Dx): Intra-abdominal abscess – due to bacteria. Unlikely other source – ie. not pneumonia or urinary tract infection (UTI).
Plan:
1. Patient currently looks well and states feeling better since the drain. Would continue antibiotics (Abx) and drain with serial Computerized Tomography (CT) to ensure adequate drainage.
2. Infectious Disease (ID) to see the length of prescription (Rx) for bacterium and suggestion for Abx.
3. Monitor Ileus – likely functional but CT scan today will help determine if there is a trans. point.
Patient: for now patient soft with no abdominal pain. Suggested fluids until he passes gas or gets hungry. Have discussion with his wife and patient.

Signed: Fenech 416-664-0300

NURSING NOTES

Date: 07/09/05
Time: 12:30

Patient ambulated using high walker accompanied by Registered Nurse (RN) and wife. Short walk to the nursing station and back to room and tolerated well. Patient resting in bed. Patient informed to be up for CT scan in 14:30 hr.

I was sent for a CT scan to see how things were going.

CT ABDOMEN REPORT

Date: 07/09/05
Time: 12:51

Physician: Reznick, Richard
Location:
Name: Glouberman, Seymour
DIS IP
MRN ft   Visit #   Sex   Age
2397544 251013277   M   65Y
Status: complete
Abdomen Computed Tomogram
Event Time: Wed, 07 Sep 05 1251
Thu, 08 Sep 05 0911 Documented by
Accession*: 301738198
Read By: David Gianfelice, MD

Date Dictated: 07Sep2005
Exam Report
REPORT (VERIFIED 2005/09/08)
CT ABDOMEN AND PELVIS

TECHNIQUE: Volumetric acquisition in the region of the abdomen and pelvis following infusion of intravenous contrast with axial and coronal reconstruction.

CLINICAL INFORMATION: Pre-anastomotic infected hematoma drainage by a percutaneous catheter evaluation.

COMPARISON STUDY: I am comparing to previous examination which dates 5 September 2005 which is the examination performed pre-percutaneous drainage. There are bilateral discrete pleural effusions which have increased slightly since the previous examination. There are atelectatic changes at both lung bases which are otherwise unremarkable.
Since the previous examination we note the appearance of a discrete-to-moderate amount of free fluid in the peritoneal cavity mostly situated in the perihepatic and perisplenic regions. There are multiple hypodense lesions at the level of the liver parenchyma unchanged from the previous examination and compatible with benign lesions. The adrenals, spleen, pancreas and retroperitoneal structures are normal. There are again noted two non-obstructed calculi at the level of the left kidney which is otherwise normal. Since the previous examination there has been placement of a percutaneous catheter in the more laterally placed fluid collection which has decreased moderately in size since the intervention. The more medially placed fluid collection remains unchanged and suggests that this fluid collection is partially organizing; this does not communicate with the percutaneous drainage catheter. There is no other significant change since the previous examination.

IMPRESSION: Placement of a percutaneous catheter has reduced the size of the more laterally placed fluid collection but has not significantly changed the more medially placed collection. This is most probably due to the fact that there is organization and loculation in this infected hematoma; a second percutaneous drain maybe helpful to complete the drainage. In the meanwhile, aggressive irrigation may in fact liquify this organized hematomoa. Appearance of disrete-to-moderate amount of free fluid in the peritoneal cavity and bilateral pleural effusions suggests that the patient may be in positive fluid balance.

CT ABDOMEN REPORT CONT'D   **Date: 07/09/05**
                             Time: 12:51

There are no new fluid collections compatible with other abscesses noted on this examination. There is however persistent small-bowel obstruction most probably due to edema at the anastomotic site. No other significant change.
PCI/E024K
Verified By: David Gianfelice, MD

During these few days, the residents were the source of information, reassurance, prognosis, and advice. They came in waves, usually in small groups, and while there, they could respond to the small worries, the twitches, the state of my bowel, the state of the infections, and the condition of my heart. I tried to get a sense of what was going on and understand how to get better. The residents represented different disciplines: surgery, of course, but also internal medicine, cardiology, and infectious diseases. They came at different times, and once the emergency was over, they seemed to stop talking to each other, so there were slightly conflicting diagnoses and prognoses that came with their visits. My heart was okay; the infection had cleared. There were no results from the culture yet. But that too would come.

As the days passed, the residents began to lose interest. One medical resident, who often came alone, seemed to be particularly bored with my case. I am still not sure why he continued to come. The others, except for infectious diseases, spent almost no time with me. I had somehow moved outside their domain of concern. All this reinforced my appreciation for the emphasis on acute conditions in hospital. It also was a practical instance of the results of specialization.

Specialists have a focused interest on a specific area and a deep understanding of it. There is a growing capacity in health care to treat clinical problems associated with ever more specific conditions. Specialization and sub-specialization in modern medicine has increased significantly since the 1950s. Warnings were issued back then that the excessive specialization could lead to a fragmentation in the care of patients. Even though the number of formal specialties was limited, partly as a result of such warnings, the growth of subspecialties has continued as more and more knowledge is gained about particular organs or diseases. Within ophthalmology, for example, there are at least two subspecialties dealing with the retina. Mount Sinai Hospital in New York proudly boasts of more than 300 clinics and programs, each of which represents a distinct medical area.

Probably the earliest specialists were the Ashipu, Mesopotamian priest doctors who believed that every organ had its own god, and illness came from angering that god. The Ashipu made the appropriate sacrifices. The modern medical joke is that the specialists have themselves become the gods of their particular organ and patients make sacrifices to them.

GENERAL SURGERY	Date: 07/09/05

Temperature (T) 38 degrees, Vital signs stable (VSS). 97% on respiratory assessment (RA). 09:20 Urine output (U/O) drained 10 units. White blood cell count (WBC) = 11. Bloated, felt very weak yesterday. Feels better now. Soft abdomen. Left Upper Quadrant (LUQ) pain. Clean wound. Drain bloody. Plan: Continue antibiotics (Abx).

Signed: Dr. Zaid Yasser

DOCTOR'S ORDER SHEET	Date: 07/09/05 Time: 14:50

Physician's Signature and Order: C. Arcarn. T/O Dr. Sahajpal/ C. Arcarn
Ceftriaxone 1gm IV every 12 hours.
Signed: C. Arcarn
EKG, CK/Troponin, Cardiology Consult, Irrigate drain with 20cc Normal Saline (NS) every 6 hours.
ASA (Aspirin) 2 tablets (81mg) po x 1 now.
IV 2/3 + Y3 + 20 illegible. 100cc/hour.
Signed: A. Sahajpal
D/C drain irrigation with 20cc NS.

CONSULTATION FORM   **Date: 07/09/05**

DATE: September 7, 2005
CONSULTANT'S NAME: B. Basarra
REFERRING M.D.: Dr. Reznick
CONSULTATION REQUESTED FROM: Infectious
Diseases (I.D.)
REASON FOR CONSULTATION: 64 year old man
with laparoscopic right hemicolectomy, anastomosis
hematoma drained. Positive fever, White Blood Cell
Count (WBC), ileus. The patient is not responding
to Intravenous (IV) Antibiotics (Abx). Please help in
diagnosis. Thank you.
Signed: Dr. Z. Yasser, PGYA

CONSULTANT'S SUMMARY:
I.D.: 64 year old man.
RFR: Mx re: Gr (-) bacilli bacteremia
Past Medical History (PMHx): Villous tumor right
colon, laparoscopic right hemicolectomy August 23,
2005 (side notes illegible).
NUDA: Meds: Heparin, Zantac, Flagyl 500", Maxiflor
400', Ampicillin 1g every 6hours.
H.P.I.: Since August 23rd successful. Post Operative Day (POD) #7 patient developed intraperitoneal
bleed, was treated and recovered. Developed small
wound infection in hospital, sent home, but on POD#4
on Keflex, returned to hospital POD#6 August 29th
with fever and small amount of abdominal pain. CT
Scan showed collection at anastomosis site that was
not drainable. Therefore, he was discharged (D/C'd)
on Abx taken by mouth (po) – Keflex x 1 week.
POD#13 Sept.5 back to Emergency Room (ER) with
rigors, chills, febrile > 39 degrees. CT Scan showed
increase in size of collection at anastomosis site.
Interventional Radiology– drain inserted for red-brown
fluid from questionable hematoma. Suggested infected hematoma as no evidence of anastomotic leak on
CT Scan (extravasation of contrast). Started on Maxi,
Ampicillin, Flagyl, on admission September 5. Blood
cultures grew G (-) Bacilli from admission.

RECOMMENDATIONS:
Now has ileus – felt weak and nauseous yesterday.
Today, much better, positive flatus and walking.
Maximum temperature during visit = 39.5 degrees
on admission; since = 38 degrees. Slight cough,
no sputum. Has positive appetite, no nausea or
abdominal pain, at rest.
On Examination (O/E): Blood Pressure (BP) 140/78,
Heart Rate (HR) 72, Temperature (T) 37.2, Respira-
tion Rate (RR) 20, Oxygen Saturation m RA 96%,
Alert and Oriented x 3.

CONSULTATION FORM CONT'D   **Date: 07/09/05**

Neuro: no nodes
Chest: Bowel Sounds (BS) throughout clear, no sounds
Cardiovascular: S, +S, no EMS, no MM, positive YYY, no edema
Abdomen: Slightly tender, BS faint, drain to right – non-tender, no nodes, midline healing, slight long flank, healing bruises
Labs:
Sept. 6, 2005:   140 / 3.8   Calcium (Ca) 2.20
11.1: 105: 371   110 / 22   Magnesium (Mg) 0.89
9.7   Illegible
0.8
Cultures:
August 29 Urine CAS (+)
September 5 Abscess/Collection (+) PND
September 5 Wound swab = Grm + illegible
September 5 Blood = Grm + bacilli – no arobic growth on plates; illegible PND on plates.
ECG: Deep increase in III and AVF? T wave down in latleads.
64 year old post intra-abdominal operation with hematoma at illegible anastomosis and superficial wound infection. Infection will likely go to hematoma +/- illegible from abdominal collection. Now illegible on current antibiotics.
RECOMMENDATIONS:
Plan:
1)   Continue current management – flagyl + Moxi flox Intravenous (IV), Ampicillin IV. Monitor clinical condition (temperature, drainage, po intake) and consider step down to po (by mouth) regimen at that time. Coverage should include anaerobes and grm (enterics likely).
2)   Repeat BW and ECG. Will D/W staff.

DATE: September 7, 2005
CONSULTANT'S NAME: Dr. Basarra

The nurses were assigned to me on a daily basis. Each morning, the staff nurse would decide who would take care of which patients, and somehow I was assigned to a different nurse almost every day that I was there. This meant that however sick I felt, I was forced to form a new relationship with the person who would be there for the next twelve hours. In every case, I worked very hard to make her know that I would only call for her if it was really necessary. The bargain was that I would try to make her life as easy as possible if she would be there when and if I really needed her. This was easy to arrange with some nurses and significantly more difficult with others. But every one of the nurses had quite intimate contact with me and did things for me that I could not do for myself. They had to bring me the urine bottle and measure the amount of urine that came out. In my chart, there are detailed accounts of the input and output measures. They all had to repack my open wound after it was examined by the surgical residents every morning. They had to empty the drainage bag attached to my tube and measure the contents. They had to take my temperature and blood pressure. They could do all this with a tender touch or not, with more or less material, and with more or less care. They came to replenish the intravenous more or less after the machine beeped. Some were friendly, while others just did their job. Friendly nurses would wave to me after I began to walk and as they went to work with other patients. My chart showed that I was cared for by fifteen different nurses over a nine-day hospital stay. The porters who took me to the various testing rooms changed each time, and even the food ladies did not remain the same. The only continuity came from an older, slightly bent over woman who always looked at the floor as she came to mop, empty the trash, and clean the bathroom. Did she speak English? She glowered silently as she went about her job.

NURSING NOTES

Date: 07/09/05
Time: 16:30-18:20

Time: 16:30
Patient's dressing changed as ID team took out old packing. Patient packed with 1/2 inch ribbon saline soaked gauze and tolerated well. Patient resting comfortably in bed. Wife at bedside. No complaints at this time.

NURSING NOTES CONTINUED

Date: 07/09/05
Time: 16:30-18:20

Time: 17:40
Patient resting in bed with no shortness of breath
(SOB), no chest pain (CP). Aspirin (ASA) 80mg x
2 by mouth (po) given as ordered. No complaints.
Wife at bedside.

Time: 18:00
Patient resting in bed. Urine Output (U/O) = 700cc.
Patient ambulated x 1. Patient refused dinner as patient doesn't like food. Pain minimal. Drain = scant
output. Wife at bedside.

Time: 18:20
Blood work collected and sent. Visual acuity (VA)
rapid and intact. Patient resting in bed with no SOB,
no chest pain (CP), and no distension noted.
Signature Illegible

Despite all the recording of medical and nursing data, no one kept track of how often I was washed or how frequently my bed was changed because these tasks were not written into the record. I was first washed after being in hospital for four days when a particularly friendly and talkative practical nurse took charge of my care. My sheets were changed after several unfortunate episodes of incontinence when my bowel began to work unexpectedly. The record does include walking (which is called "ambulation"). Perhaps if we found Latin terms for bathing and changing beds then these activities could also be recorded. I supported myself on a walker and was accompanied by Susan and a nurse for my first circuit around the nursing station – once around on the first day and twice around the next day with Susan alone. After four days in hospital, I had a bowel movement – greenish black stuff. And I was once more allowed to eat and was taken off the IV antibiotics and given tablets.

The nurse manager of the ward came to visit and asked how I was finding the care. I complained that there was little continuity in the nursing care: I had had a different nurse for almost every shift. She was very sympathetic and said that she understood what I was saying. She was new to the job and would have a meeting with the staff nurses to determine what could be done about changing the priorities a bit to keep the same nurse for a longer stretch. Even though this was a short-stay surgical unit, there should be some continuity of care for individual patients. Our conversation made no difference: the nurses kept changing. As I got better, the nurses became noticeably less able. I guessed that they gave the most skilled nurses to the sickest patients. I wondered how much authority the nurse manager has to change this seemingly fundamental way of working.

This industrialization of health care has been happening for a long time. The process began when the analysis of work developed by Frederick Taylor was applied to nursing. Taylor believed that one could break down factory work into a series of discrete atomic tasks that could be more easily performed by supervised, relatively unskilled workers. Nursing work has been studied for years using time and motion studies derived from Taylor. The result has been a growing reduction of nursing into the tasks that are required in the care of patients with particular conditions. Nurses' "skills" include the tasks that they can perform well. And the nurse managers assign nurses with the appropriate "skill mix" to patients as needed. As patients get better, fewer "skills" are needed. Continuity of care is not part of this calculation. Making sure that the unit is covered with an appropriate "skill mix" is what the head nurse must worry about.

NURSING NOTES

Date: 07/09/05
Time: 19:30-23:50

Time: 19:30
Patient received in bed, awake, alert and oriented x 3. Left peripheral intravenous (PIV) at 2/3, 1/3 and 20mg potassium chloride (KCl) at 100ccc/hr maintained. Abdomen soft and slightly distended. Bowel sounds (BS) faint to left (L) quads. No normal saline intravenous (NIV) and flatus.

NURSING NOTES CONTINUED

Date: 07/09/05
Time: 19:30-23:50

Right drain in situ with sero-sang drainage. No edema.
Will monitor.
Signature Illegible

Time: 21:30
Patient incontinent of stool.

Time: 23:50
Ativan 0.5mg g/L given.

DOCTOR'S ORDER SHEET

Date: 07/09/05

Physician's Signature and Order:
Medical consult to see: Serum Cholesterol, Triglyantes (fasting in the a.m.). Change Ceftriaxone to every 24 hours. 2 D echo. Repeat ECG in the a.m. Repeat CK/ Troponin test in the a.m.
Date and Time Ordered: 07/09/05 @ 21:15
Ativan 0.5mg – 1mg SL Q HS PRN, Discontinue (DC) Zantac.
Pepcid 20mg IV BID --- REFUSES, T.O. Dr. S. Punnen
Signature Illegible
Medical Consults. Aspirin 81mg. Repeat Troponin test done in the a.m.
Date and Time Ordered: 07/09/05 @ 22:30
V/O Dr. Punnen/ Signature Illegible
Disregard Pepcid order.

I was visited on a daily basis by the surgical residents, who checked the wound; by residents from internal medicine, who seemed bored, did not do very much, and came around out of diminishing curiosity; by cardiology residents, who checked my heart and wondered if I might have had some kind of heart related event (they would follow up); and by residents from infectious diseases, who told me that I most likely had had septicemia and that chills and shaking or "rigors" often accompany the high fever associated with this kind of infection. They were culturing the blood that had been retrieved from the abscess. Septicemia! That's pretty serious. I was gradually assimilating the notion that there had been a very real possibility of death.

Thursday, September 8, 2005

Thursday September 8, 2005
From: Misha Glouberman
Sent: Thursday, September 08, 2005 1:44 AM
To: Friends Family And Colleagues of Sholom Glouberman
Subject: Update
September 8 2005
Hello,

To let you all know – after having been sent home the weekend of the 27th, my father has been readmitted to the Toronto General Hospital as of a couple of days ago. It seems that there are some infections resulting from the surgery. It is likely that he will be in the hospital for a few more days, as the doctors treat and monitor the infections.

My understanding is that these sorts of infections are not unusual following colon surgery. While the effects of the infection are stressful and unpleasant, the doctors assure us they are no great cause for concern. My father continues to receive excellent care and has many visitors along with the constant attention of my mother.

As always, I'll keep you updated on future developments, and am glad to pass on any emails to my father.

- Misha

CONSULTATION FORM   **Date: 08/09/05**

CONSULTATION REQUESTED FROM: General Surgery

REASON FOR CONSULTATION: Cardiology

CONSULTANT'S SUMMARY:
64 year old man referred with ECG. No sign of Chest Pain (CP) or Shortness of Breath (SOB). Already seen by Medical Consult in this regard (see note). Villous illegible for right colon August 27th. Complicated by Gram Negative Bacterium (grm) and retroperitoneal bleeding. CRF HTN, former smoker. Very active – swims 2 miles a day.

CONSULTATION FORM CONT'D   **Date: 08/09/05**

On Examination: Heart Rate (HR) 60, Blood Pressure (BP) 150/80.

Chart checked.

Cardiac (N) S.S, no sims negative, JVP 2 cm, ASA (Aspirin).
Abdomen slightly distended.
ECG post operation (post-op) illegible, LVH
September 5 – Sinus rhythm today now deep Q was infused? illegible

September 7 – Sinus rhythm, nonspecific T-waves Δ's troponin illegible.
Chest x-ray (CxR) – Normal (N)

Seeing 64 year old man = complicated post-op course. No symptoms of cardiac. ECG Δ's nonspecific and may be due to rate and read placement. No further work up (W/U) for cardiac needed unless patient develops cardiac symptoms. Recommended for follow-up (F/U) = MD re BP control.
Signing off – Marc Allen.

DATE: September 8, 2005

CONSULTANT'S NAME: Marc Allen

CONSULTATION FORM   **Date: 08/09/05**

REFERRING M.D.: General Surgery

CONSULTATION REQUESTED FROM: Medical Consult

REASON FOR CONSULTATION: Non Specific T-wave changes.

CONSULTANT'S SUMMARY:
64 year old man who was told on July 29th that he had high blood pressure (BP) – (170/90) but was not treated at the time of Pre-Operative assessment.
DM / increase in cholesterol/ (+) family history of CAD (Mother/87).
Had laparoscopic right hemicolectomy on August 23rd, 2005 for villous polyps – went back home August 27th, 2005. Came back to Emergency Room (ER) on August 29th with wound infection which was open and started on Keflex x 7 days – finished yesterday.

CONSULTATION FORM CONT'D   **Date: 08/09/05**

CT on the 29th showed leak and hematoma around anastomosis. General Surgery's concern is that he had non specific T wave infection. Previous shortness of breath (SOB), Normal Sinus Rhythm (NSR). Never had previous chest pain, or any symptoms and was told that he has acid indigestion and is relieved by Zantac. He had illegible flu and was told by his family physician that he had some non specific ECG changes and had stress test – Normal (N) – and his ECG came back to NSR.

Past Medical History (PMHx):
1) Ex-smoker illegible.
2) DM/ increase in cholesterol
- PHx (+) CAD for Mother
- Social History: Occasional drinker, quit smoking

Prescriptions:
1) Flagyl
2) Moxiflox
3) Ampicillin
4) Aspirin

On Examination:
- Sleeps comfortably in bed.
- Illegible
- BP 140/65, Heart Rate (HR) 65, Respiration Rate (RR) 14
Cardiovascular and Respiration (N)
Gastrointestinal – illegible
Treatment (Tx):
Blood Culture: illegible.
Complete Blood Cell Count (CBC): 121 illegible.
P/t 471 / PT = 14.71 / INR 1 11
Troponin test < 0.2
Na = 1401   K = 331 Cl = 110 Mg = 0.29
AST = 10 ALT = 12 / ALP = 61

Impression:
Seems that there are no acute cardiac changes. The non specific ECG changes could be related to his bleeding/infection.

Recommend:
1) Stick with Aspirin 81 mg po every 3 hours x 3 days.
2) Repeat his cardiac enzymes / in hospital and as an outpatient and to be followed up by family physician.
3) Will continue to see him and see his team with staff

Signature Illegible.

105

CONSULTATION FORM CONT'D   **Date: 08/09/05**

(Staff) RECOMMENDATIONS:
1) ECG Δ's non specific. No evidence of MI/ACS.
2) Patient complained of melena last night. Observe
   for UGIB especially since he is on ASA (Aspirin).
   Δ Zantac, and illegible.
3) Outpatient – exercise, stress test by family MD
   when patient is on to R/O CAD.
4) Outpatient follow-up re high blood pressure.

CONSULTANT'S NAME: M. Otremba

NURSING NOTES   **Date: 08/09/05
                       Time: 02:00-06:00**

Time: 02:00
Ativan 0.5 mg g/L given.

Time: 06:00
Patient asleep.

GENERAL SURGERY   **Date: 08/09/05
                       Time: 06:30**

Temperature (T) max = 38, T current = 37.2, Pulse
(P) = 75 – 96, Respiratory Rate (RR) = 20, Blood
Pressure (BP) = 157/70 – 160/81, Urine (U) =
3200/2400, Drain = 50ml/24hrs.
Afebrile, Vital Signs Stable (AVSS). 98% in Re-
spiratory assessment (RA). Urinary output (U/O)
1700/12hrs. Drain 50. Bowel Movement (BM).
Troponin test negative. Patient feeling well. Walked
yesterday. Less distended.
Plan: Clear fluids (CF) – Diet as tolerated (DAT)

Signed: Dr. Zaid Yasser

CLINICAL NOTES   **Date: 08/09/05
                       Time: 07:15-23:45**

Medical Staff: Please see note on "yellow" sheets.
Signature illegible.

Time: 07:15-12:00
Received patient in bed. Alert and oriented x 3.

CLINICAL NOTES CONTINUED

Date: 08/09/05
Time: 07:15-23:45

Vital signs stable (VSS)-Afebrile. Peripheral intravenous (PIV) of 2/3 and 1/3 with 20 potassium chloride (KCl) at 100mg/hr infusing well. Chest clear,
no shortness of breath (SOB), no chest pain (CP).
Abdomen soft and non-tender. Bowel sounds (BS)
x 4 present and flatus. Abdominal dressing changed
by Registered Nurse (RPN) with scant drainage
of sero-purulent. Right drainage in situ with scant
drainage. Patient ררדvoids adequate amount using
urinal. No edema. Wife at bedside. Patient currently
resting in bed watching TV. Will monitor. Patient
ambulated in the hallway x 2 accompanied by wife.
Signature Illegible

Time: 12:15
Patient's wife came to nursing station informing
nurse that patient told medical consultant that he
passed black stool last night but wife stated she
didn't think it was black. Order written by doctor for
stool. Will follow.
Signature Illegible

Time: 16:00
Patient resting in bed with no complaints. Stool for
occult blood collected and sent.
Signature Illegible

Time: 18:20
Patient resting in bed. Urinary output (U/O) adequate. Patient ambulated x 1. No voiced concern
throughout the shift.
Signature Illegible

Time: 20:00
Patient received ambulating around hallway with
wife. When patient returned to room vital signs
stable (VSS). Patient complained of nausea. Gravol
– 50mg intravenous (IV) given. Abdomen soft and
bowel sounds (BS) present. Patient passing flatus
and having bowel movements (BM). Dressing intact.
Right drain in situ with sero-sang drainage noted.
No edema. Will monitor.
Signature Illegible

Time: 22:00
Patient states nausea better. Will monitor.
Signature Illegible

Time: 23:45
Patient complains unable to sleep. Ativan 1 mg
sublingual (SL) given.
Signature Illegible

DOCTOR'S ORDER SHEET   **Date: 08/09/05**

Date and Time Ordered: 08/09/05
Physician's Signature and Order: Dr. Z. Yasser
Clear Fluids – Diet as Tolerated (CF-DAT). Cardiolo-
gy Suggestions: D/C (discontinue) cardiac enzymes.
Signature Illegible

Date and Time Ordered: 08/09/05
Physician's Signature and Order: Signature Illegible
RN, Dr. Z. Yasser
Medical Consults: Stool for occult blood. D/C Zantac
and start illegible. Continue monitoring Complete
Blood Cell Count (CBC). Aspirin 81mg by mouth
(po) and follow-up (F/U) by his family physician
(F/P) regarding stress test and Blood Pressure (BP)
prescription (Rx) if necessary.
08/09/05 @ 20:15
Chart Checked.
Infectious Diseases (I.D.) Suggested: Amox–Clav
500/125 tablet po times daily (TID), total 14 days
treatment (tx). Can D/C Intravenous (IV) Antibiotics.

Signed: V. White RN, Dr. Z. Yasser, Signatures Illegible.

Friday, September 9, 2005

I was sent for an echocardiogram. This seemed like a
second adventure into unknown and very strange territory
to me. This time, I was received by a surreal high priestess of
echocardiography. Her name was Lay Chain Wong, according to the chart. I was ushered into the ceremony of echocardiography, and as its priestess, Dr. Wong carried herself with
ceremonial dignity and grace. She said almost nothing as
she led me into a small dark room with many monitors and
lots of twinkling lights. Would she read my fortune? Would
she tell me what the future held in store? Would it be life or
death? I learned nothing.

No riddles, no pronouncements – only barely spoken
instructions. I was a supplicant, converted to this sorcery. I
would do whatever I was told. I was entranced by the lights.
She hooked me up to the test machinery.

"Lift your arm." And I was hooked up to many wires; the lights kept flashing.

"Lie back." And I felt as though this was the serious investigation. We would find out the truth.

"Breathe." And I breathed.

"Don't breathe." And I stopped and held my breath.

I had no idea what an echocardiogram did, but it seemed to be about the technologist obtaining visions of the heart. I later found a description on the internet:

An echocardiogram is a test in which ultrasound is used to examine the heart. The equipment is far superior to that used by fishermen. In addition to providing single-dimension images, known as M-mode echo that allows accurate measurement of the heart chambers, the echocardiogram also offers far more sophisticated and advanced imaging. This is known as two-dimensional (2-D) Echo and is capable of displaying a cross-sectional "slice" of the beating heart, including the chambers, valves and the major blood vessels that exit from the left and right ventricle.

For a resting echocardiogram (in contrast to a stress echo or TEE, discussed elsewhere) no special preparation is necessary. Clothing from the upper body is removed and covered by a gown or sheet to keep you comfortable and maintain the privacy of females. The patient then lies on an examination table or a hospital bed. Sticky patches or electrodes are attached to the chest and shoulders and connected to electrodes or wires. These help to record the electrocardiogram (EKG or ECG) during the echocardiography test. The EKG helps in the timing of various cardiac events (filling and emptying of chambers). A colorless gel is then applied to the chest and the echo transducer is placed on top of it. The echo technologist then makes recordings from different parts of the chest to obtain several views of the heart. You may be asked to move from your back and to the side. Instructions may also be given for you to breathe slowly or to hold your breath. This helps in obtaining higher quality pictures. The images are constantly viewed on the monitor. It is also recorded on photographic paper and on videotape. The tape offers a permanent record of the examination and is reviewed by the physician prior to completion of the final report.

Here are the results:

ECHOCARDIOGRAM REPORT	**Date: 09/09/05** **Time: 09:18**

GLOUBERMAN, SEYMOUR 2397544
University Health Network
Height (cm): 178
Weight (kg): 84
BSA: 2.04
Rhythm: Sinus
Gender: M
Status: Inpatient
Hospital Loc: 9 ES
Study Quality: fair
Study Type(s): 2-D Echo/Doppler (00001)

Indications: Assess LV size and systolic function.
Ischemic ECG changes.

Left Ventricle: The left ventricular chamber size is
normal. Mild concentric left ventricular hypertrophy
is observed. Minimal hypokinesis of the left ventricle
is observed with regional variability (EF 50-59%).
The basal inferior and mid inferior wall segments
are hypokinetic.

Right Ventricle: The right ventricular cavity size is
normal. The right ventricular global systolic function
is normal.

Aortic Valve: The aortic valve is trileaflet. The aortic
valve leaflets are mildly thickened. There is no
evidence of aortic stenosis. The AV peak gradient
is 25mmHg. The AV mean gradient is 10 mm Hg.
Mild to moderate aortic regurgitation is present. The
aortic regurgitation is posteriorly directed.

Mitral Valve: The mitral valve leaflets are slightly
thickened. There is mild mitral regurgitation observed. The mitral regurgitant jet is posteriorly
directed. Mitral annular e1: 0. Urn/sec.

Tricuspid Valve: The tricuspid valve leaflets are
morphologically normal. There is trace tricuspid
regurgitation present. The Right Ventricular Systolic
Pressure is calculated at 36mmHg.

Pulmonic Valve: The pulmonic valve appears normal
in structure and function.

Left Atrium: The left atrium is mildly dilated.

Pericardium: There is no pericardial effusion.

Aorta: There is mild dilatation of the ascending
aorta.

I was taken back to my room. I was told that I had no abnormal heart condition, although how I was informed later became an issue. The echocardiogram had found that there was some regurgitation in some of the valves in my heart. I never saw the report until I retrieved the record, and even then, I didn't really examine it in any detail. When I had another echocardiogram a year later, I was told that this mild regurgitation, though not serious, meant that I should take prophylactic antibiotics before I had may teeth cleaned. At the time while I was in hospital, I remained blissfully ignorant of my leaky valves – I had been told that I was okay. I felt that recovery could begin again in earnest.

GENERAL SURGERY   Date: 09/09/05

Afebrile, Vital signs stable (AVSS). Urinary output
(U/O) 1700/shift. Drain scant. Feeling well. Slight
epigastric pain. Passing gas. Abdomen soft.
Plan: Encourage ambulation.

Signature Illegible

INFECTIOUS DISEASES REPORT   Date: 09/09/05

64 year old man with post op anastomosis leak/
bleed – collection drained.
- Patient doing well. Eating, bowel movements,
  flatus, ambulating.
- Afebrile x 2 days. Temperature (T) max 37.9 de-
  grees this a.m. Patient feels well.
- Blood pressure (BP) 160/70, Heart Rate (HR) 66,
  Oxygen Saturation 98% Respiratory Assessment
  (RA). Chest clear. Abdomen soft, non-tender, no
  evidence of wound infection (clear, healing well).

Blood Culture: Bacteroides Fragilis   88: 7.2: 342
137/105: 3.4/26 (82)

Anastomosis collection: Bacteroides Fragilis
Plans: Patient is improved on intravenous (IV)
antibiotics (Abx). Culture shows anaerobic growth
(bacteroids) which is covered by flagyl. Still at risk of
other organisms given source site.

ID REPORT CONTINUED   **Date: 09/09/05**

Therefore, suggest step-down to the antibiotic
Amox-Clav by mouth (po) 500/125, as patient tolerating oral intake.
General surgery to determine follow-up (F/U) with
respect to imaging/collection status?

Signature Illegible

NURSING NOTES   **Date: 09/09/05**
                                       Time: 12:15-20:30

Time: 12:15
Received patient lying in bed awake, alert and oriented x 3. Wife staying in room with husband. Vital
signs stable (VSS), T 37.9 (oral). Chest expansion
symmetrical. Fine crackles auscultated. Decrease in
air entry (A/E) bases bilateral. Incentive spirometer
(I/S) deep breathing and coughing, and ambulation
encouraged. Abdomen soft, distended, Bowel sounds
(BS) x 4, flatus, no bowel movement (BM) yet today.
Abdomen dressing (midline) dry and intact (D+I). Left
(L) multipurpose drain site satisfactory with sanguineous returns. Patient voiding in bathroom (BR) and
urinal. (L) Peripheral intravenous (PIV) 2/3 and 1/3 +
20 potassium chloride (KCL) infusing at 100cc/hr. Site
satisfactory. Patient to echocardiography (echo) at
09:00. Patient ambulating in hallway using low walker
accompanied by wife at 11:00. Plan to get patient in
shower today and ambulate.
Signed: Beth McCallum RN

Time: 17:00
Patient resting in bed. Wife at bedside. Patient went
to shower with assistance from RPN earlier this
afternoon. Abdominal dressing changed and wound
cleaned. Cleaned with N/S and packed with 1/4 inch
ribbon gauze normal saline (NS) soaked. Covered
with 2x2 hypofix. Patient tolerated well. No voiced
concerns at this time.
Signed: B. McCallum RN

Time: 18:40
Patient ambulating in hallway accompanied by wife.
Voiding well in urinal. No voiced concerns at this time.

Time: 20:30
Patient at 19:20 - Vital signs (VS): Temperature (T)
37 degrees, Respiration (R) 20, Pulse (P) 70, Blood
Pressure (BP) 140/68, Oxygen saturation 97% Respiratory Assessment (RA). Patient alert and oriented.

NURSING NOTES CONTINUED

Date: 09/09/05
Time: 12:15-20:30

Chest clear. Incentive spirometer in use and encouraged, bowel sounds present. Abdomen soft, slightly distended, flatus present, stated BM today. Patient voiding in urinal clear amber. Abdominal dressing dry and intact (D+I), drain dressing D+I, and drain draining scant serosang. PIV infusing 2/3 and 1/3 with 20 KCI. Slight edema present in upper/lower extremities. Patient denies any pain, nausea or dizziness. Wife in room and patient up walking.

DOCTOR'S ORDER SHEET

Date: 09/09/05

Date and Time Ordered: 09/09/05
Physician's Order and Signature: V. White RN
Chart Checked -- HHD -- Checked at 20:25 hours.

Saturday and Sunday, September 10 and 11, 2005

NURSING NOTES

Date: 10/09/05
Time: 00:30-05:00

Time: 00:30
Patient asleep.

Time: 3:00
Patient asleep. Complained of nausea, Gravol given.

Time: 05:00
Patient asleep.
Signature Illegible

GENERAL SURGERY

Date: 10/09/05
Time: 06:45

Patient awake, no complaints. Afebrile, Vital Signs Stable (AVSS), blood pressure (BP) 155/70, urinary output (U/O) 4955 in 24 hrs, drain 10cc. Bowel movement (BM).Had some abdominal pain with taking the antibiotics (Abx). Echocardiograph (echo) okay, no concerns. Belly soft.
Plan: Will continue with Abx and water.
Signature Illegible

Time: 08:30
Received patient in bed awake, alert, oriented x
3. Wife staying overnight with patient – present at
bedside. VSS. 02 Saturation 97% respiratory assessment (RA). Chest expansion symmetrical. Chest
clear on auscultation. Decreased air entry (A/E)
bases. Incentive spirometer (I/S) encouraged and
ambulation encouraged. No complaint of chest pain
(CP) or shortness of breath (SOB). Abdomen soft,
non-tender, slightly distended. Bowel sounds (BS)
increased (+) x 4. Flatus but no BM today. Patient
voiding in urinal clear amber. Abdominal dressing dry
and intact (D+I), drain dressing D+I. Right drain scant
serosang returns. Peripheral pulses present (ppp).
No complaint of leg pain, slight edema to extremities.
Left (L) Peripheral Intravenous (PIV) 2/3 and 1/3 20
KCI infusing at 100cc/hr. Site satisfactory. Pain score
2/10. Patient reports having abdominal pain last night
after receiving antibiotic. Did not report to night RN.
Patient states that he told team doctors on rounds this
morning. Pain not present at this time.
Signed: B. McCallum RN

Time: 09:00
Patient complained of nausea 25mg Gravol by mouth
(po) given.
Signed: B. McCallum RN

Time: 10:00
Nausea still present Gravol 25mg po given.
Signed: B. McCallum RN

Time: 11:30
Intravenous (IV) – saline lock (S/L): Abdominal dressing changed for discharge on 2x2 serosang on ribbon
gauze. Wound clean, no odours, redness or swelling
around site. Wound bed pink and moist. Cleansed
with normal saline (N/S). Packed with N/S soaked 1/4
inch ribbon gauze covered with 2x2 and hypofix. Dr.
Jadad from eHealth innovation is family friend. Doctor was in to see patient updated.
Signed: B. McCallum RN

Time: 12:30
Patient up in chair in hallway. Linens changed by
RPN. Patient completed morning care in bathroom
(BR) independently. Patient complained of some
nausea still but no Gravol given at this time.
Signed: B. McCallum RN

Time: 16:15
Temperature (T) 38 degrees (oral) at 14:00. Will continue to monitor and will notify Dr. Orzech.

NURSING NOTES CONTINUED
Date: 10/09/05
Time: 08:30-19:15

Patient has no nausea or vomiting (N/V) at this time. No complaint of pain. Patient states feeling well today. No other voiced concerns.
Signed: B. McCallum RN

Time: 17:20
T down 37.2 degrees (oral). Wife relieved that T down.
Signed: B. McCallum RN

Time: 19:15
Patient resting in bed. Wife at bedside. Voiding large amount of clear urine in BR. Left (L) saline lock (S/L) flushed and patent.
Signed: B. McCallum RN

I like hospital food. I have worked in one hospital or another for the last 25 years and am always surprised at how I have learned to eat institutional food with some pleasure. At Baycrest, where I go every day, the food is Kosher-Caribbean. The patients are Jewish and most of the kitchen staff and many care staff are Caribbean. A special favorite is chicken gumbo soup. Other kosher Caribbean specialties include sweet and sour flanken, and occasionally, kosher jerk chicken. At the Toronto General, the porridge was excellent (probably because of the hospital's Scottish heritage). The lunch of turkey and mashed potatoes with cranberry sauce was scrumptious, and the butter tart that came with it was of gourmet quality. I was hungry and feeling good for the first time in weeks. Our friends the Perlitzes brought Chinese food. We gobbled down what we could and stuffed the rest into the small unit fridge.

DOCTOR'S ORDER SHEET
Date: 10/09/05

Date and Time Ordered: 10/09/05
Physician's Order and Signature: V. White RN
Chart Checked at 10:40. SL Intravenous (IV) TO/Du
T.O. Dr. Hujuh/ V. White RN. SL IV

DR.'S ORDER SHEET CONT'D   **Date: 10/09/05**

Date and Time Ordered: 11/09/05
Physician's Order and Signature: Checked at 20:00
hours.
Signed: Dr. Merino

Date and Time Ordered: 10/09/05
Physician's Order and Signature: B. McCallum V.
White RN, Signatures Illegible.
Checked at 21:15 hours. Anusol suppository 1/2 tab-
let up to G x 1 day as needed (PRN). Colace 100mg
po bid. Illegible 30cc po bid until bowel movement
(BM).

CLINICAL NOTES   **Date: 11/09/05**
Time: 03:00-15:00

Time: 03:00
Patient asleep.

Time: 05:00
Patient asleep.

Time: 06:40
Patient awake, reading, no complaints. Blood Pressure (BP) 150/70, Pulse (P) 75, Temperature (T)
37.2 degrees, T max 38 degrees yesterday, 96%
R/A, Urinary Output (U/O) 2300/24 hrs.

Time: 07:15-13:10
Late entry. Received patient at 07:30 hrs feeling
awake and alert. Vital signs stable (VSS), afebrile.
States he feels better today. Shower given with
minimal assistance and tolerated well. Abdominal
dressing showed wound healing well. Minimum
sero-sang drainage soiled – 1/4 inch ribbon gauze
soaked with normal saline (N/S). Reapplied. Multipurpose drain remains in situ draining scant sero-
sanguineous discharge. Patient fully ambulatory.
Family at bedside.
Signed: Marian Garcia.

Time: 15:00
Patient stated had bowel movement (BM) today.
Does not want colace this evening. Patient requesting annusol support for hemorrhoids. Patient self-
administered suppository. No other voiced concerns
at this time.
Signed: B. McCallum RN

116

Susan's brother Chaim came to visit. He was astonished that Susan had stayed in the hospital every night for the whole week. He urged her to leave, if only for a while. He stayed with me while she went home for a bath.

The weekend was otherwise uneventful. I walked and increased the number of circuits to four. There were visits by everyone. Lots of friends now could come to visit. Our friends Keith Oatley and Jenny Jenkins came by with a wonderful collection of obscure magazines. I began to read *New Grub Street.* I watched the end of the American Open Tennis Championships on television. I held forth for other visitors. I continued to eat the delicious food.

I enjoyed the visits, got tired, slept, and walked around the nursing station. I still was not very strong, but I was much more optimistic. I weighed myself on the hospital scale and found that I had lost twenty pounds since the surgery.

CLINICAL NOTES   Date: 11/09/05
                                  Time: 17:00-21:30

Time: 17:00
Resting with no complaints. Afebrile.
Signed: M. Garcia

Time: 18:30
Resting in bed with wife at bedside. No complaints.
Signed: M. Garcia RPN

Time: 21:30
At 19:20 Vital signs (VS): T 37 degrees, R 20, P 82,
BP 138/60, Oxygen saturation 97% RA.
Patient alert and oriented. Chest clear and audible.
Incentive spirometer in use, bowel sounds present.
Abdomen soft and slightly distended. Abdominal
dressing dry and intact (D+I) + p/c + drain D+I,
drainage scant serous-sang. Patient resting in bed-
room, had BM today, slight edema present in upper
and lower extremities. Peripheral pulses present
(ppp). Patient denies any pain, nausea, dizziness.
Wife by patient's side.

NURSING NOTES
Date: 11/09/05
Time: 21:30-23:50

Time: 21:30
At 19:10 Vital Signs (VS): T 37 degrees, Respiration
(R) 20, Pulse (P) 78, Blood Pressure (BP) 138/70,
Oxygen saturation 97% respiratory assessment (RA).
Patient alert and oriented. Chest clear and audible.
Encouraged use of incentive spirometer (I/S) and
deep breaths and encouragement, bowel sounds
present. Abdomen soft and slightly distended, flatus
present, no bowel movement (BM) today. Voids well
in bathroom. Abdominal dressing dry and intact (D+I)
with ptc-tube scant serous sang in bag. Saline Lock
(S/L) peripheral pulse present (ppp). Slight edema
in upper/lower extremities. Patient denies any pain,
nausea or dizziness. No signs of shortness of breath
(SOB) or chest pain, within room. Patient up walking.

Time: 23:50
Patient awake. VS taken, T 37.2. Ativan given.

Monday, September 12, 2005

NURSING NOTES
Date: 12/09/05
Time: 00:20-06:00

Time: 00:20
Patient asleep.

Time: 3:00
Patient asleep.

Time: 5:00
Patient asleep.

Time: 6:00
Patient asleep and voiced no concerns.

GENERAL SURGERY
Date: 12/09/05
Time: 07:00

Temperature (T) max 38 degrees; T lowest 36.5
degrees, Blood Pressure (BP) = 142 – 170/ 69 – 84
c = 142/74, Pulse (P) = 60 – 80, c = 82, Respiratory Assessment (RA) = 97%, Afebrile, Vital Signs
Stable (AVSS) on RA, Drain = scant. Patient doing
fine. Eating by mouth (po). No issues.

NURSING NOTES
Date: 12/09/05
Time: 08:00

Time: 08:00
Received patient awake in no distress. Refused
to take colace and heparin (anticoagulant). Small
dressing to right side of abdomen dry and intact
(D+I). Pain score 2, vital signs stable (VSS), Oxygen Sat 97%. Wife slept over last night. She is also
anxious about patient's care and condition. Request
annusol suppository.

DOCTOR'S ORDER SHEET
Date: 12/09/05
Time: 09:00

Date and Time Ordered: 12/09/05 @ 09:00
Physician's Signature: Signature Illegible.
Please measure urine output (accurate I+O).¬¬¬¬¬
¬¬¬¬¬¬¬¬¬¬¬¬¬¬¬¬ Medical Consult Suggestions:
Will Sign Off, Thanks – Signature Illegible

MEDICAL CONSULT
Date: 12/09/05
Time: 09:30

MED Consult: 64 year old man post op Left (L)
Hemicolectomy. Last seen for Electro Cardiograph
(ECG) - non-specific T waves. Started on ASA. Currently asymptomatic. Last ECG done Sept. 7. Can
follow up with family MD and arrange stress echocardiograph (echo). Call us if you have concerns or
new issues arise
Signed: M. Quteri Resident 3 (R3)

On Monday, Dr. Reznick appeared. He was all smiles. He
looked at the wound. He asked how I felt. The drainage bag
had now been empty for a day. My temperature was down. I
had had a bowel movement and was on solid food. I was still
pretty weak.

"You are improving very quickly and I think that you
will be able to go home tomorrow. I know that you've been
through a lot this past week, so we'll keep you in until then

just to be sure. From what I can tell, we will never really know where the infection came from, but that is not unusual. Why don't you get dressed this afternoon and take a break from the hospital. You can take your wife out for a coffee to a café in Yorkville. She has been so devoted to you, and you are well enough to take the afternoon off. Get away from the hospital. You must be good and tired of this place. In fact, why don't you go to Yorkville and buy her a gold bracelet to show her your gratitude. For now, let me take a look at your wound and the tube."

He took off the bandages and looked at the wound.

"It's healing very well. I think we can safely take out the tube right now."

"Right now?" I quaked. "How will you do it? Does it need some anesthetic?"

I liked the tube. It put me in touch with Tapski. It was both odd and pleasing to me that an upper-class Englishman should be given such a Russian-sounding, even a possibly Jewish nickname.

"No, we just pull it out and cover it with a bandage. It's quite simple." He called for the nurse to prepare to bandage the opening and pulled the tube. A bit of fluid came out with it. Then the bandage covered it and it was done. Reznick left.

I was now completely free of appurtenances; except for the open wound, I had no attachments, no holes. Susan and I decided that Yorkville was a bit beyond my capacity, but perhaps we could go downstairs for a Tim Horton's cup of coffee. I decided to practice by taking a few circuits around the nursing station.

The second time around, I felt something wet on my side. I looked down and saw a pink splotch on my bathrobe that was growing at an alarming rate. I opened the robe and saw that the bandage was soaked through and was oozing a pink fluid that had gone down my side to my underpants.

Had the tube been blocked and was this more pus escaping? Was this bleeding caused by extracting the tube? What was going on?

CLINICAL NOTES

Date: 12/09/05
Time: 13:00-13:30

Time: 13:00
Dr. Reznick removed drain. Small dressing applied. No drainage at present.

Time: 13:30
Patient called. Very upset. Afraid drain site leaked lots of sero-sang fluid; explained that this is normal.

I went to the nursing station and told them that I was leaking fluid. "Please come immediately to stop it, to redress the opening – to do something to stem the leak." I went back to my room and my less-skilled nurse came quickly to redo the bandage. She put a bigger bandage over the opening to absorb the fluid, but that soaked through in a matter of minutes. I returned to the desk and found the more senior nurse who had put on the initial bandage with Dr. Reznick.

"What's going on here?" I asked. "I was supposed to go to Yorkville."

"Don't worry," she said. "It sometimes happens that when a tube like that is withdrawn, some fluid from your body cavity escapes. It is not blood or pus and is nothing to worry about."

"Do you realize how frightening it is when something like that happens without warning?" I asked. "And it is continuing to leak," I complained. "This is really unacceptable. I was told to go to Yorkville...as if there was nothing like this that could happen."

"I'm sorry that it happened to you, but it is very rare," she said. She attached a plastic bag with a spigot to the hole, and I was back with attachments. I asked for a private meeting with the resident when she came to the unit that afternoon. I went back to my room.

The cleaning lady was there; she broke her silence. She said, "You had better wash the bathrobe. That stuff stains and you'll never get it out if you don't do it right away. I'll get you some soap."

Susan and I were both extraordinarily grateful for this oddly sympathetic and quite human advice. It was as if she understood at some much deeper level our anxiety and how to do something about it. Susan washed the bathrobe and hung it in the bathroom.

I frantically read *New Grub Street*. The infectious diseases resident came by on his daily visit. "Hi, we got the results of the blood culture. It turns out that the blood that was extracted by the radiologist was infected with an anaerobic bacillus called bacillium fragilis. That was the cause of your septicemia. These bacteria are normally in the gut, but must have leaked out after the colon resection. The antibiotic we gave you is effective for it and should stop the risk of re-infection."

INFECTIOUS DISEASES CONSULT   **Date: 12/09/05**

64 year old man post right hemicolectemy anastomosisomic leak/heatoma causing bacteroides infection. Patient well. Up in chair. (+) Eat, (+) bowel movement (BM). Tolerating medication by mouth (po). Temperature (T) max over the weekend 38.1 degrees. Patient states no concerns though. 2D echo shows no variations.
Blood Pressure (BP) 142/72, Pulse (P) 66, Oxygen Saturation 97% Respiratory Assessment (RA)
- Drain discontinued this a.m. by General Surgery Staff. Plan to possible discharge (d/c) patient tomorrow.

Plan: Continue antibiotics (Abx) for total course of 14 days. Provided team happy with control. Will review with staff and ask the General Surgical team to call if any concerns.

Signed: Basarra

"When did the results come?" I asked.

"They were on your chart this morning."

Did pulling the tube increase the chance of re-infection?

That afternoon, Dr. Choi came to the room. I asked to see her; I wanted to present the catalogue of my complaints. Everything from her misinformation to Reznick's failure to forewarn me of a possible leak was on my mind. I was upset, yet I worried about how to present these complaints to her. I did not want to embarrass her, yet I wanted her to understand what I was upset about.

"You have been very attentive in many ways," I said, "always there when we phone, always available to deal with difficulties. I appreciate your intelligence. However, what made you think that when you opened the wound, it would heal in two weeks? You have looked at it every morning now for almost a week and it is now ten days since you opened it. Do you really think it will be completely healed in the next four days? You must understand how devastating it was when the home-care nurse told me the next day that it would take six to eight weeks to heal.

"Today I was told by the surgeon that we would probably never know what the source of the infection was, but later the infectious diseases resident came by and told me that the results were put in my chart this morning before he came. Now I must say that I am worried that pulling the tube may have been premature and that some infection might remain in the fluid that leaked all over me. Is it really true that such leaks are so rare?"

"Look I'm sorry that all these things have happened," she replied. "I will talk it over with Dr. Reznick." She was not at all embarrassed. I was yet once more being excessively delicate. I felt foolish. I resolved to discuss this with Dr. Reznick myself.

CLINICAL NOTES

Date: 12/09/05
Time: 16:00-21:45

Time: 16:00
Ostomy bag applied to drain site, leaking lots of sanguineous fluid.

Time: 18:00
Temperature (T) 37 degrees – eating and drinking well. Asked to empty ostomy bag. Patient sitting with friends. Answered that "it's only a little bit of fluid in bag?"

Time: 18:30
Had Chinese food for supper.

Time: 20:00
Received patient in bed reading. Wife at bedside. Afebrile. Oxygen saturation 98% in respiratory assessment (R/A). Abdomen soft. Bag over right drain site in situ with same pinkish drainage voiding well.

Time: 21:45
Up and ambulated in hallway with wife.

DOCTOR'S ORDER SHEET

Date: 12/09/05

Date and Time Ordered: 12/09/05
Physician's Signature: Signature Illegible
Annusol to cream/ointment. V.O. Dr. Reznick.
Checked at 21:00 hours.

Tuesday, September 13, 2005: Discharge

NURSING NOTES

Date: 13/09/05
Time: 01:00-08:00

Time: 01:00
Voiding well. Urinal emptied.

Time: 03:30
Sleeping.

Time: 06:00
Awake. Medication Taken. Voided well.

NURSING NOTES CONTINUED

Date: 13/09/05
Time: 01:00-08:00

Time: 08:00
AVSS. Dressing to abdomen intact, no oozing. Abdomen soft, bowel sound present. Bag to drain site in place. Small amount of sero-sang drainage in bag. No complaint of pain.

Dr. Reznick arrived on Tuesday morning.

"Many patients need to be jostled and pushed out of being sick," he said. "I have to be very optimistic with them so that they don't fall into a depression. You've had a really bad time. It happens, and I thought that you could use a little push. So I suggested the coffee outside. The leak doesn't really mean anything and it usually doesn't happen when you pull a tube. But you are now basically ready to go home. We will do a few more tests and send you on your way. You'll come back and see me on September 23 to make sure that everything is okay."

I was eager to get home and in no mood now to deliver my list of complaints. Susan was still worried that I would have to come back yet again. I finished reading *New Grub Street*.

GENERAL SURGERY

Date: 13/09/05

Afebrile, Vital Signs Stable (AVSS) 2250cc. Patient slept well. Soft abdomen, clean incision. 50-75cc, scent coming from drain site. Plan: Computerised Tomography (CT) scan today. +/- drain. May discharge (d/c) home today or tomorrow.

Signed: Dr. Yasser

NURSING NOTES

Date: 13/09/05
Time: 10:00-12:00

Time: 10:00
Up, showered; wife assisted. Managed well.

NURSING NOTES CONTINUED

Date: 13/09/05
Time: 10:00-12:00

Time: 10:30
Abdomen dressing packed with normal saline (N/S) soaked salvage 1/4 inch wound tissues; pink around edges; healing.
Signed: J. Cleary RN

Time: 12:00
Patient for CT scan @ 13:30
Signed: J. Cleary RN

A new CT scan was in the works to see what was happening in my gut. This visit to the scanner was memorable in a new way. I was brought down to the scan waiting area, and there was a patient in one of the closed rooms with a sign that marked him as possibly suffering from a communicable infectious disease. We were parked opposite the door when it opened and he was wheeled out to the general area. Those accompanying him were masked and gowned. We were not. They left him there while they arranged the next stage of investigation. We moved to another part of the open area with some fear and in self-defense. They kept moving the infected patient in and out of the side room at irregular intervals.

After about half an hour of waiting, Susan asked the clerk when my scan would occur.

The new clerk said, "It's all in the computer and they will call you when they are ready. As you can see, it's quite busy." We waited, and in about fifteen minutes, the scan technicians emerged from yet another door.

"Am I next?" I asked. "We have been waiting for almost an hour."

"Who are you? You don't show up on the computer, so we didn't know that you were here. But now that you ask, we will fit you in before the next patient."

Fifteen minutes later, I had the scan and was brought back to my room by a porter.

CT ABDOMEN REPORT

Date: 13/09/05
Time: 13:30

Physician Reznick. Rich
Location: DIS IP
Name: Glouberman, Seymour
MRN #   Visit #   Sex Age
2397544 251013277 M   65Y
Abdomen Computed Tomogram
Event Time: Tue, 13 Sep 05   1330
Wed, 14 Sep 05   1146
Documented by
Accessions: 301744432
Read By: David Gianfelice, MD
Date Dictated: 13Sep2005
Exam Report:
REPORT (VERIFIED 2005/09/14)
CT ABDOMEN AND PELVIS

TECHNIQUE: Volumetric acquisition in the region of the abdomen and pelvis following infusion of intravenous contrast followed by axial and coronal reconstruction.

CLINICAL INFORMATION: Percutaneous drainage of abscess recently; the catheter has been removed.

COMPARISON STUDY: I am comparing to previous examination which dates the 7 September 2005. Since the previous examination the percutaneous catheter in the right lower quadrant has been re-moved. The bilateral minimal pleural effusions have almost completely resolved. There is only a small amount of residual fluid in the peritoneal cavity. The liver is unremarkable with the exception of multiple hypodense lesions compatible with simple cysts which are unchanged from the previous examination. The spleen, adrenals, pancreas and retroperitoneal struc-tures are normal. There is again noted an exophytic cyst at the left kidney and a non-obstructed calculus in the mid portion of the right kidney also unchanged from the previous examination. In the lower abdomi-nal and pelvic region we note that the percutaneous drain which is situated in the more laterally situated collection has been removed. The laterally situated collection has completely resolved. The medially situ-ated collection which most probably represents an or-ganized hematoma which maybe secondarily infected has reduced in size since the previous examination and now measure 4.7 x 3.3 cm as compared to 6.0 x 5.1 cm on the previous examination. The hetero-genicity in the fat around the anastomosis has also significantly decreased which suggests at least partial resolution of the inflammatory disease in this region.

CT ABDOMEN REPORT CONT'D	Date: 13/09/05 Time: 13:30

Examination in the pelvic region is unchanged from previous. There is no evidence of new fluid collections in this region.

IMPRESSION: There is a residual fluid collection in the peri-anastomotic region which may require percutaneous drainage if the patient is febrile. This collection has however diminished in size since the previous examination and if there is no febrile illness there, this may suggest that there will be spontaneous resolution of this collection with time. There is overall decreased inflammatory response in the peri-anastomotic region, almost complete resolution of the free fluid in the peritoneal cavity and significant resolution of the bilateral pleural effusions.

Verified By David Gianfelice, MD

The scan showed that the abscess was considerably smaller. The radiological intervention seemed to have cleared it. There was another smaller blood ball, but it would disappear on its own. I was now capable of showering myself and could walk around the nursing station two or three times at a go, and I did this at least twice a day. I had read *New Grub Street*, so I was capable of reading more than magazines and thrillers.

I visited the surgical nurse again and she reorganized home care. Once the results came that afternoon, we took a taxi home.

NURSING NOTES	Date: 13/09/05 Time: 14:00

Patient d/c'd home via wheelchair accompanied by wife. No complaint of pain or discomfort. Teaching given concerning prescriptions and Dr.'s follow-up appointment. Patient appears happy and comfortable upon d/c.

DOCTOR'S ORDER SHEET

Date: 13/09/05
Time: 18:00

Date and Time Ordered: 13/09/05 @ 18:00
Physician's Order and Signature: Dr. Z. Yasser
CT Scan today. Discharge (D/C) home with Home
Care and prescriptions. Follow-up (F/U) in 1 week
with Dr. Reznick.

Signature Illegible

I wanted to work hard at recovery. I walked outside the first day back and set up my room upstairs again. I expected to take some time to recover but began to get in touch with people at work again.

Wednesday, September 14, 2005: Home Care

Rachelle returned in the morning. She welcomed me back and said that she would be moving the next day, which was her normal day off, and that she would be back on Friday. She now had lots of sticks and swabs and ribbons to work with and declared that the wound had improved during the time I was in hospital. That night, a substitute nurse called to say that she would be there the following morning.

Thursday, September 15, 2005

On September 15, Misha wrote his last email.

Sent: Thursday, September 15, 2005 4:27 AM
Subject: Home from the hospital
Hi.
My father is back home after several days in the hospital.
The fevers and other symptoms he had been experiencing were due to a blood infection (septicemia) by bacteria (bacteroides fragilis) resulting from the surgery.
 He is pretty tired, but also okay. He'll be away from work for the next few weeks as his recovery continues.
    - Misha

I woke up to get my wound dressed by the nurse who was covering for Rachelle's day off. The woman who came was lovely and proceeded to tell us that we did not have the right kind of equipment to dress the wound properly, but she had some things in her car that would do it. She would be away until Saturday; in the event, she returned on Sunday.

Over the next five days, until Rachelle had safely moved house, five different nurses came. Each was a lovely woman. Each was a caring person. Each had more stuff in her car. And each had her own idea about how to dress the wound properly. Each put on a different kind of bandage over the dressing, and each thought that her way was best. The wound healed well, but the other result was severe irritation around the bandage; the skin became red and bloody after the series of new "best" bandages were applied.

I was called by the quality assurance coordinator of the Community Care Access Centre (CCAC), which had commissioned the work through a private home nursing agency. "How was the care delivered to you by your home care nurse?" I was asked. I told her that the nurses were without exception wonderful people who each did a terrific job, but that I was most dissatisfied with the fact that they appeared to change on a daily basis while my primary nurse was gone. This fragmentation of care seemed to be just as bad for community nursing as it was in the hospital.

I guess that the quality assurance person in the CCAC must have gotten in touch with the nursing agency because the next day, I received a call from their quality manager who asked me what I thought of the care that I was getting. Did I like the nurses? Were they on time? Did they listen to me? Were they customer focused enough? I was forced to repeat my concerns. I reassured her about the quality of the individual nurses. In fact, I was surprised at how good they all were, how attentive and eager to do their jobs well. However, I would prefer to have fewer: "Great care, lousy continuity."

She then put me in touch with the manager of the service and encouraged a face to face meeting to work through these problems in earnest. The service manager called and wondered what was wrong with Rachelle; she was one of their best, after all. What was I dissatisfied with about her care? Would I like to change nurses? I was still pretty tired, but ready to keep talking. I told her that Rachelle was a spectacular nurse. I always eagerly awaited her arrival. My wound was being well cared for. I just felt that there were too many different nurses caring for me when Rachelle was off. She lost interest at that point and thought that we should have a telephone meeting to sort it all out. She delayed this for the next six weeks until my wound was healed. We never spoke again. I did not pursue it either. So much for continuity of complaint.

The whole process became more and more funny and irritating at the same time. Here were these perfectly capable women being managed in a way that fragmented their work and made it more difficult for patients yet probably suited the time management needs of the agency.

Before the end of this second week out of hospital, the Infectious Diseases resident called and asked if I could come in for a follow-up visit. I arranged a visit to Dr. Adrienne Chan on September 23, the same day I was to see Dr. Reznick.

Friday, September 23, 2005: Follow up Visit to Dr. Reznick

I thought that I would unburden myself to Dr. Reznick when Susan and I went to see him on September 23 about what had gone wrong with the surgery. I wanted to communicate some of the rather complex feelings I had about how my care had been managed. We came to the outpatient department and were soon shown into an examining room where the nurse unwrapped the open wound. Dr. Reznick came into the room, looked at the wound, and pronounced that it was healing well. I too was healing well: no fever, beginning to behave more normally. I had almost completed the course of antibiotics and should stop taking them once they had run out. I was relieved to hear that I would be free of medication soon. The results of the biopsy were in and showed no signs of cancer. This was an enormous relief for Susan especially, who had worried mightily about this. I somehow had not really ever thought that I might already have cancer. I'm not sure why.

PATHOLOGY REPORT   **Date: 23/09/05**

UNIVERSITY HEALTH NETWORK
Toronto Medical Laboratories
Department of Pathology

Toronto General Hospital
200 Elizabeth Street
Toronto, Ontario,M5G 2C4
Tel: 416-340-3325

Patient Name: Glouberman, Seymour
Copath #:S05-19323
MRN: 2397544
Service: Surgical Service
Collected: 23/08/05
DOB: 10/10/40 (Age: 64)
Visit #: 251010054
Resulted: 31/08/05
Gender: M
Location: ES8 GEN S
HCN:4433950088
Facility: TG
Ordering MD: Reznick, Richard K.
Surgical Pathology Consultation Report

SPECIMEN(S) RECEIVED
1. Intestine-Lg Res: rt.colon

DIAGNOSIS
Right colon, a short segment of distal ileum and an appendix, right hemicolectomy:
- Right colon with tubulovillous adenoma, low grade, 4.5 cm in diameter and free resection margins.
- Negative for high grade dysplasia or malignancy.
- Appendix and ileum, within normal limits,
- Eighteen lymph nodes identified and negative for malignancy (0/18).

PATHOLOGY REPORT CONT'D   **Date: 23/09/05**

ELECTRONICALLY VERIFIED BY: Runjan Chetty,
MD dtk/8/31/2005

CLINICAL HISTORY none given

GROSS DESCRIPTION

1. The specimen container labeled with the patient's
name and as "right colon" contains a hemicolectomy
specimen received in 10% buffered formalin. The
terminal ileum measures 5.5 cm in length x 4.2 cm
in circumference, the cecum measures 7.5 cm in
length x 7.0 cm in circumference, the colon measures 15.8 cm in length x 8.9 cm in circumference.
The appendix measures 7.3 cm in length x 0.6 cm in
diameter. On gross examination, there is presence
of a polypoid-like tumor on the proximal aspect of
the colon, measuring 4.5 x 3.0 cm with a 0.8 cm in
luminal height. The tumor is 3.2 cm away from the ileocecal valve, 8.5 cm away from the distal resection
margin and 7.5 cm away from the proximal resection
margin. The tumor is tan in colour and appears to
be submucosal in nature. The appendix is tan in
colour and appears to be grossly unremarkable. The
mucosal surface of the terminal ileum and cecum appears to be grossly unremarkable. No other nodules
or polypoid-like tumor is identified on the cut surface
of the colon. Within the fatty tissue, multiple lymph
nodes are identified grossly ranging in size from
0.2 x 0.2 to 0.6 x 0.2 cm. Representative sections
submitted as follows:

1A - proximal resection margin, perpendicular section with India ink

1B - distal resection margin, perpendicular section
with India ink

1C-H - representative section of the polypoid-like tumor

1I - representative section taken of the ileocecal valve

1J - representative section taken of the cecum
mucosa

1K - representative section of the terminal ileum
mucosa

1L, M - representative section of the colon mucosa

1N - representative section from the appendix

1O - five lymph nodes

1P - five lymph nodes

1Q - three lymph nodes

1R - five lymph node

I asked about diet, and Dr. Reznick said that I could
eat anything I liked: taking out a mere eight inches of colon
made no real difference to digestion. Finally, I asked about

the implications for Misha and wondered about a genetic test for susceptibility to colon cancer. He said he would put me in touch with people at Mount Sinai who could do the genetic testing.

Susan asked if I now wanted to speak to him alone. But it seemed to me that with all this good feeling, I could discuss how I was treated while she remained in the room. I said, "I'd really like to talk to you about the care I got while I was in hospital."

"Sure," he said and smiled.

I am not very confrontational at the best of times and I was no longer sure of what I wanted to raise. I retreated in my mind to a discussion of the fragmentation in the system of care, how the various players had not really spoken to each other so that the coordination of my care was quite fragmented. This was not really what I wanted to talk about. I wanted to get out of there as fast as I could. So it seemed that it was the best I could do at the time.

He said that I was unlucky and that in about 3% of cases, things went wrong in this way. He was sorry that it had happened to me and that was all there really was to say. My comments about the system and the fragmentation of care were perceptions that came from my analytic perspective, but did not really reflect on what had happened to me.

He left. The nurse returned to repack the wound. She may have sensed some of my disappointment and proceeded to unburden herself. She said, "I've been working here for many years. I'm almost ready to retire. I like it here, but keeping the doctors happy is a lot of hard work. I do what I can, but I'm getting too old for this."

I felt as I had the last time before the unnecessary enema: I had lost my stuffing and could not properly say what was on my mind. I have thought a lot about what else I could or should have said. I guess that this whole long story about my operation has been my attempt to say it all. Here once more was this great disparity between what I knew and how I could make myself understood.

(After getting the medical record with the entire pathology report, I realized that I had not only had a piece of colon removed, but my appendix was also taken out. It seems odd to me that no one ever mentioned this, though some of my friends thought that the appendectomy was an irrelevance).

We left for our follow-up appointment with the Infectious Diseases department and found Dr. Adrienne Chan, who brought us to a small, windowless office decorated with what looked like a massive number of safari souvenirs – jungle animals of all kinds. It seemed to be an allusion to the more exotic diseases faced by the Infectious Diseases group. Later, we discovered a giant stuffed lion in the waiting room. I was not sure if this was to cheer up patients, to declare the royal nature of the service, or to urge upon us an informality that was not really there.

I did not like taking the very strong antibiotics. They made me feel slightly sick, and I felt that this was another delay in getting back to "normal." I hoped that this would be the last visit with Dr. Chan and I could get on with my recovery. It was not to be.

"I don't think you should go off the antibiotics just yet," she said. "Your last CT scan showed that there is still a blood ball near your colon and it might contain more infected blood. I would like to do another scan soon to make sure that that blood ball has disappeared before you go off the antibiotics. I will give you a renewable prescription for two more weeks and we will schedule a CT scan as soon as possible."

It was scheduled for Friday, September 29. She wrote to Dr. Reznick.

INFECTIOUS DISEASES REPORT   **Date: 23/09/05**

NAME: Glouberman, Seymour
DOB: 10Octl940
MRN: 239 7544   G
VISIT #: 254441422
LOCATION: 5304-AMS-Infectious Diseases
Date Dictated: 23Sep2005
Dr. Adrienne Chan, Dr. Nick Daneman, Dr. Jan
Hajek, Dr. Vanessa Allen, Dr. Susy Hota, Dr.
Sharmistha Mishra, Dr. Darrell Tan
Toronto General Hospital,
Dr. Richard Reznick Department of Surgery TGH

Dear Dr. Reznick:
RE: Sholom Glouberman MRN 2397544
I saw your patient, Sholom Glouberman, in follow
up. He is a 64-year-old gentleman who had Bacteroides species bacteremia secondary to an abscess
in his abdomen following colectomy for a villous
adenoma. From September 5-13, 2005, he was
treated with intravenous ampicillin, moxifloxacin and
metrinidazole, and from September 13 until today he
was "stepped down" to oral Clavulin. Subjectively,
Mr. Glouberman is doing quite well with no fever or
systemic symptoms. He still has some fatigue.

A repeat CT scan on September 13, 2005, showed
an interval decrease in size of his collection.
My plan is for him to continue on Clavulin, given that
there is a residual 4 x 3 cm collection. The duration
of antibiotic therapy will be determined by his clinical
status and based on repeat imaging, which I have
ordered.

Yours sincerely,

Adrienne Chan, MD Infectious Diseases Fellow

Wayne Gold, MD, FRCPC Infectious Diseases
Consultant

Report Type: Letter
Date Released: 20Feb2006
Date Transcribed: 23Sep2005
Transcribed By: DJV

Chapter Four

Further Complications:
Effects of Surgery or Aging?

Thursday, September 29, 2005: Visit to the ER

I was still working hard at getting better. I decided to grill some steaks on our backyard barbecue. Barbecuing is a sign of good health and would be a renewal of my masculine prowess. I noticed that our grape vine had taken over much of the area near the barbecue and decided to do a bit of weeding while I waited for the steaks to cook. I pulled at the vine and fell backward, tumbling down a small incline and hitting my calf against a rock. In a bit of shock, I got up to see if I had hurt anything. Not much pain. I shook my leg and brought the steaks into the house. Susan and I ate while my leg began to hurt a bit.

After dinner, Marvyn Novick, an old friend of mine, came to visit, and I sat in a corner of the sofa as the pain in my leg became worse. I tried desperately to ignore it and succeeded for a while.

"Go to the hospital to check it out," Susan said.

"No way," I replied. "I've had enough of hospitals. It will get better on its own."

When Marvyn left, the pain got worse, and I grudgingly consented to call Telehealth Ontario, a service that allows callers to present their symptoms to a registered nurse who will offer advice on what to do next. I described what had happened and the nature of the pain, and the nurse concluded that this was worth a visit to the ER for an X-Ray to determine if the leg was broken. So off we went for our third visit to the emergency room in as many weeks. We arrived at eleven p.m. and they knew us.

"Hello," said the doctor, "I remember you from last time."

"Hello," said the nurse. "Welcome back. We will have your leg X-Rayed in no time."

The orderly placed me in a wheel chair and said, "I'll get you there." He wheeled me to the X-Ray unit and brought along another patient as well – a young man with a gunshot wound that was acting up. Ah, the romance of the ER.

The X-Ray technician was angry. She said to all of us, "You're not supposed to be here."

The orderly gave her the order and said that it was late and he wanted to get me to X-Ray so that I could get home and not have to wait forever.

She grudgingly agreed to do it.

I was wheeled back to my cubicle, and the doctor arrived about fifteen minutes later and said, "No break. It's probably a torn muscle in your calf. It is very painful and will take about a week to heal."

DEM NURSING ASSESSMENT	Date: 28/09/05 Time: 23:59

DEPARTMENT OF EMERGENCY MEDICINE
NURSING ASSESSMENT

Present Complaint: Fall

Triage Assessment: Complained of right calf pain, difficulty bearing weight. Blood Pressure (BP) 15/79, Pulse (P) 75-78, Oxygen Saturation 98% on R/A.

Past Medical History: FTW; Discharged (D/C) 2 weeks ago – August 23/05 for colon resection (benign).

Allergies: None Known

Medications: Yes – Amo-Clav

Method of Arrival: Ambulatory

Accompanied By: Wife

Assessment Obtained From: Signature Illegible

Triage Nurse Signature: Signature Illegible

Primary Nurse Signature: Signature Illegible

DEM ASSESSMENT CONT'D	Date: 28/09/05 Time: 23:59

Initial Vital Signs Left Arm: Supine: BP 15/75, P 78,
Respiration Rate (RR) 18
A)   Neurologic:
B)   Cardiovascular: Regular Pulse, no skin abnor
       malities, Skin warm.
C)   Respiratory: Rhythm regular, depth adequate,
       quality adequate.
D)   Abdominal: N/A
E)   Genitourinary: N/A
F)   Musculoskeletal: Calf Pain
G)   Spine & Pelvis: N/A
H)   Head & Neck: N/A

Nurse's Signature: Signature Illegible

ES REPORT	Date: 29/09/05 Time: 00:30

EMERGENCY SERVICES (ES) REPORT
DEMOGRAPHICS
Brought In By: Family Member
ALERT
Presenting Complaint: Fall, Right Leg Injured
Time: 00:30
Physician's Name: David Carr
Triage and Acuity Scale: Urgent
DISPOSITION
Discharge Diagnosis: Right Calf Muscle Injury
Attending MD: Signature Illegible

CLINICAL NOTES
-   64 year old man fell 18:30 today while pulling
     weeds. Ambulating with difficulty.
-   Puritus – colon resection - benign
-   Post op August 23, 2005 for benign colon
     resection.
-   Re-admitted Sept. 5-14 for sepsis (abdominal).
-   Right Leg and tender calf
-   No swelling atrophy.
-   Peripheral Pulse Present (PPP)
-   Ra knee/ankle
-   Troponin test negative
-   Illegible
X-Rays Ordered: X-ray
E.D. Interpretation: Right Tibula/Fibula

Signature: Signature Illegible

We went home well after midnight.

Friday, September 30, 2005: CT Scan

The next day, I was back at work in the morning and in the hospital for the CT scan in the afternoon. I was now in the outpatient part of the imaging department. Several women were waiting for CT scans that would tell them how their cancer was doing. I was chastened by the contrast between our states. I was told that I would get the results the following Wednesday. I drank the contrast fluid and had the test.

CT ABDOMEN / PELVIS REPORT   **Date: 30/09/05**
Time: 15:00

```
MRN #      Visit          Sex   Age
2397544   251013277   M     65Y
Physician: Reznick, Rich
Location    Name
DIS IP        Glouberman, Seymour
Status: supplemental
Abdomen Computed Tomogram
Event Time: Fri, 30 Sep 05  1500
Accession*: 301758808
Read By: Zeinab Layton, MD
Date Dictated: 30Sep2005
Exam Report:
REPORT  (VERIFIED 2005/10/03)
CT ABDOMEN AND PELVIS
```

TECHNIQUE: Volumetrically acquired unenhanced axial images of the abdomen and pelvis were obtained with 5-mm collimation.

COMPARISON STUDY: 13 September 2005

CLINICAL HISTORY: Follow up abscess. Right hemicolectomy for villous tumour.

FINDINGS: There has been interval improvement in the right pericolonic collection which now measures 2.6 x 2.3 cm on image #85 compared with 4.9 x 3.4 cm. There is minimal stranding in that region and the ileocolic anastomosis is intact. There is no free air and the free fluid has resolved in the interval. The remainder of the bowel and mesentery is unremarkable. There are multiple hypoattenuating lesions in the liver which are unchanged. The spleen, pancreas and adrenals are unremarkable.

CT REPORT CONTINUED

**Date: 30/09/05
Time: 15:00**

There is a well-defined round cystic lesion directly lateral to the right kidney which might represent an exophytic cyst but a clear fat plane is delineated between it and the adjacent right kidney. Given its presence in the vicinity of the previous collections, the possibility of a fluid collection rather than an exophytic cyst must be considered. It measures 3.7 cm on the current study and is unchanged from the previous. There are two non-obstructing calculi in the mid portion of the left kidney, the largest of which measures 6 mm.

There is no significant adenopathy.

There has been interval resolution of the small bilateral pleural effusions. There are tiny nodules noted in the right lower lobe on image #11 and in the left lower lobe on image #41 which were not discernible on the previous study likely due to obscuration from atelectasis. There are no aggressive bone lesions.

Wednesday, October 5, 2005: Bad Leg

I worked hard at making the leg better. I was working for half days. I walked a bit more each day and felt much better. I asked my medical friends for advice. Murray Enkin, the retired obstetrician, said, "Take Tylenol. Walk through the pain."

I heard from Dr. Chan. The CT scan showed that there was still a small blood ball attached to the colon, so I would have to continue the antibiotics for three more weeks.

Saturday, October 8, 2005: Worse Leg

I walked through the pain but re-injured the leg; that night, the pain was even more intense than it had been the first time. Now it was much slower to heal. My other medical friend, Dan Perlitz, said, "This can be permanent. You should go to a physiotherapist."

143

Monday, October 10, 2005: 65th Birthday

My birthday came on Canadian Thanksgiving in 2005. I wanted to celebrate turning 65 in some special way – by going to a fancy restaurant, for example – but I was in no condition to do this. In fact, I began to organize my life around permanent leg pain. I could go to work but made sure that I did not walk too far and injure my leg even more.

Thursday, October 14, 2005: CT Scan

I was given another CT scan to see if the blood ball had disappeared. By this time, I was an expert at preparing for the scan: I knew what to do and felt comfortable at the clinic.

CT ABDOMEN / PELVIS REPORT	Date: 14/10/05 Time: 18:00

Name: Glouberman, Seymour
Location: DIS OP
MRN ft   Visit #   Sex   Age   Physician
2397544   253158089   M   65Y   Reznick, Rich
Abdomen Computed Tomogram Event Time: Fri, 14 Oct 05
Read By: Zeinab Layton, MD
Date Dictated 17Oct 2005
CT OF ABDOMEN AND PELVIS
CLINICAL HISTORY:
Follow-up abscess. Patient is status right hemicolectomy for villous tumour.
PREVIOUS: September 30, 2005.
TECHNIQUE: Helical acquisitions were obtained of the abdomen and pelvis, post-IV and oral contrast administration.

FINDINGS: Adjacent to the surgical anastomosis there is a small amount of soft tissue attenuation (image 76), measuring 1.8 x 1.2 cm. There is no drainable fluid collection appreciated. There is persistent thickening of the lateral conal fascia, unchanged from previous. There is perinephric stranding, unchanged from previous. Well defined cystic lesion is again seen in the right perinephric space adjacent to the mid pole of the right kidney. This likely represents an exophytic renal cyst, however, it can be reassessed at time of follow-up.

CT REPORT CONTINUED	**Date: 14/10/05** **Time: 18:00**

The remainder of the study is unchanged from previous.

OPINION: No drainable pericolonic collection. Soft tissue changes in the adjacent pericolonic fat likely postsurgical in nature.

Wednesday, October 19, 2005: Infectious Diseases

A call from Dr. Chan told me that I was now clear and could go off the antibiotics. I took the last pill and stopped the next day. All through this time, my bowel movements were not normal, but once I stopped the antibiotic, they returned to normal in several days. I began to think I could see the end of the operation. At the same time, the open wound had now almost closed. It took almost eight weeks for it to heal. Rachelle would pay her last visit to me on October 23.

Thursday, October 20, 2005

I was booked for a follow up meeting with Dr. Reznick. I was to visit his clinic at three o'clock in the afternoon. I knew where his clinic was, and so once I heard the part of the message from his assistant that confirmed the appointment, I erased the message. We went to the outpatient clinic at the appointed time, but no one knew where Dr. Reznick was. Finally, someone told the clerk that his clinic was across the road on Thursdays. It took another ten minutes to find the number there and tell them that I was in the wrong place. I refused to walk for fear of hurting my still painful leg, and ten minutes later, a porter arrived with a wheel chair. He led us into the dungeon of the hospital and through a tunnel to cross the street. We went through endless corridors and several elevators before we reached the clinic. Once there, I waited for half an hour for Dr. Reznick to appear.

He said, "My assistant says that she told you we would be here. The staff on the other side of the road has access to my pager, so they should have contacted me immediately. I am not sure why this all happened, but they will hear from me."

I said that I must not have heard the message from his assistant. My leg also made it impossible for me to walk that much.

I told him that we had gone to the Infectious Diseases doctor after our last visit with him when he had told me to stop the antibiotics. The CT scan ordered by infectious diseases had in fact shown that a blood ball remained, and at their suggestion, I had instead stayed on antibiotics until October 20.

He said that all that was a reasonable way to proceed. He then examined me. He looked at what remained of the wound and saw that it had healed. He said that I had obviously had a very bad time and that it was most unusual for so much to go wrong on one procedure. He then looked at my calf to see what was wrong with it. My sense was that he wanted to apologize for my bad time and to make it all better.

CLINICAL NOTE   **Date: 20/10/05**

UNIVERSITY HEALTH NETWORK
Princess Margaret Hospital
610 University Avenue,
Toronto, Ontario M5G 2M9
Health Records Services
* * * CHART COPY * * *
NAME: Glouberman, Seymour
DOB: 10Octl940
MRN: 239 7544 P
VISIT #:   254402346
LOCATION: PMH Gastrointestinal Oncology
Date Dictated: 20Oct2005
Date of Visit: 20Oct2005

Mr. Glouberman is a gentleman who had a colonic tumour. He underwent a right hemi-colectomy using a laparoscopic technique.

CLINICAL NOTE CONTINUED

Date: 20/10/05

This was complicated by a postoperative bleed and subsequent peritoneal hematoma that subsequently required drainage percutaneously. He at one point had some systemic sepsis that was treated with antibiotics. He has been out of the hospital now for a good four to six weeks. He is off all antibiotics. Serial CT scans showed complete resolution of his hematoma and abscess. He feels well and is back to normal activity.

His recent hemoglobin was 117 g/L. His recent CT scan of a few days ago was normal looking to me. He feels well.

I answered several questions today. I have told him that he needs another colonoscopy in about nine months. He is going to call Dr. Rawling in that regard. I expressed empathy that he had this post-operative complication but was grateful that he was improving and getting back towards normal.

Dictated by: Richard K. Reznick, MD, MEd, FRCSC, FACS
Professor of Surgery, University of Toronto
Department of Surgical Oncology
Tel: 416-340-4137
Fax: 416-595-9846
E-mail: richard.reznick@utoronto.ca
DICTATED BUT NOT READ 2014383/407793
Transcribed by: IN
Report Type: Clinic Note
Date Transcribed: 20Oct2005

November 2005: Patient Satisfaction

In November, although there was still some pain in my leg and I feared long walks, I did go to Quebec to give my talk to the annual convention of public health doctors. I even swam in the Chateau Frontenac pool. I had a wheelchair to take me to the plane and back to my car at the end of the trip. I did the same later that month when I went to England for my semi-annual visit to work with the National Health Service. I managed both trips without too much walking and without any further incident.

I received a package from the Hospital that asked me to fill out a patient satisfaction survey. The questions on it had little to do with my experience.

In fact, the survey had almost nothing about how the different groups of people who were caring for me talked to each other. Did they "Always," "Sometimes," "Seldom," "Hardly ever," or "Never" talk to each other or listen to what the other had to say? Everyone was kind, personable, and intelligent. But many had no idea of what the others were doing or even thinking. As a good citizen, I filled it out and sent it back. Here are my responses, as recorded by the surveyors:

How were you admitted	Planned admission
Organization of admission process	Very organized
Waited too long to go to room	No
Explained reason for wait in going to room	No Valid Answer
Courtesy of admission	Excellent
One Dr in charge of care	Yes
Dr answered questions understandably	Yes, always
Dr discussed anxieties/fears	Yes, somewhat
Confidence/trust in Drs	Yes, sometimes
Drs talked in front of you	No
Courtesy of Dr	Very Good
Availability of Dr	Fair
Overall Dr care	Good
Nurse answered questions understandably	Yes, sometimes
Nurse discussed anxieties/fears	No
Confidence/trust in Nurses	Yes, sometimes
Nurses talked in front of you	No
Courtesy of Nurses	Excellent
Availability of Nurses	No Valid Answer
Dr/Nurse explained things differently	Yes, sometimes
Enough say about treatment	Yes, somewhat
Family talked w/Dr enough	Yes, somewhat
Amount of Info given to family	Right amount
Ease of finding someone to talk to	Yes, somewhat

Got bathroom help in time............................ Didn't need help

Minutes for help after call button...........................1-5 minutes

Wait time after call button reasonable...............Yes, somewhat

Explained test results understandably...............Yes, somewhat

Scheduled tests/procedures were on time.......Yes, sometimes

Treated you w/respect/dignity.........................Yes, sometimes

Had pain..Yes

Pain severe/moderate/mild..Moderate

Requested pain medicine...Yes

Minutes taken to get pain medicine.......................1-5 minutes

Did everything to control pain.............................Yes, definitely

Amount of pain medicine received......................Right amount

Discussed purpose of home meds...................Yes, somewhat

Discussed medication side effects...................Yes, somewhat

Discussed danger signals to watch for.............Yes, somewhat

Discussed when to resume normal activities.....Yes, somewhat

Family had enough recovery info..No

Knew who to call w/ questions..Yes

Received all services needed...........................Yes, somewhat

Overall care received...................................No Valid Answer

Rate how Dr/Nurses worked together...............................Poor

Would recommend for stay.............................No Valid Answer

Overall quality of food...Excellent

Condition of room/hospital environment.....................Excellent

Nurses acted on suggestions about care............................No

Found educational materials/programs................................No

Felt someone was in charge of care.................Yes, somewhat

Amount of relief from pain medication.....................Somewhat

Amount of relief from other therapies...............Did not receive

Rate health..Excellent

Days illness/Injury kept you in bed.........................Four Days

No. of times in hospital overnight/longer..........................Twice

Highest education completed............................Post university

Who completed survey...Patient

I was given a small space for verbal comments. According to the electronic survey company, I wrote, "The survey does not capture the difficulties with my hospital stay. It says almost nothing about the fragmentation of care. Individuals were all dedicated + kind and smiling, but the system did not provide adequate continuity (unreadable). Bad survey CC: President, VP nursing, VP medicine."

I also paid my bill for nine days in a private room.

December 2005: Montreal Visit

We began to plan our annual New Year's Party to celebrate my recovery.

My leg was now almost back to normal, and I could walk quite far without pain. We traveled to Kitchener on December 21 for an early Christmas celebration with our son's in-laws and then we drove to Montreal on December 23. On Christmas day, we had dinner with Susan's family at Kevin and Marcie Pask's house. Afterward, I was up all night with diarrhea. The next day, we visited our friends Ruth and Jerry Portner for lunch, then went to Susan's cousins, the Franks, for dinner.

Monday, December 26, 2005: Emergency Room Again

At dinner, I began to feel quite sick and faint and left the dinner table. I asked Marcie's daughter Violet to get Susan because I was not feeling well. When Susuan came into the room, I said that I was feeling quite faint and fainted. When I revived, I found that I had had an uncontrolled bowel movement. I went to the toilet and had a violent diarrhea attack. When Susan's cousins gave me new clothes, I returned to the living room and proceeded to faint several more times. It was decided that I would go to the emergency room at the Jewish General Hospital.

Susan called Misha, who was also in town, and asked him to come. Ruthy and Jerry Portner joined us when they learned what had happened. Here I was in the emergency room yet again.

In the ER, the nurse came into my cubicle and said, "Oh they are driving me crazy. These patients keep calling me and I have so many others to see. I'm really tired and I have to be here all night. It looks like it is going to be a rough night."

"I'm a pussy cat," I offered. "I will make your life as easy as pie. I am not demanding and I will be nice to you. Just cross me off your list of difficult patients."

She smiled and walked off.

The doctor came and took my history, several blood samples, and decided that I was dehydrated from the diarrhea. The doctor was about to go off duty, but a new doctor would be there during the night. He thought that they should take a stool sample because I might be infected by the C. Difficile bacteria. He explained that such bacteria could thrive when a post-surgical patient was on antibiotics for a long time. He would rehydrate me with three units of saline solution and take a stool sample. The nurse returned and smiled and attached me to an intravenous drip-set to speedily pump the saline into me over several hours.

Hershey and Esther Frank left when the Portners came, and soon Misha also left when it became clear that I was feeling much better.

They asked for a stool sample to culture. I went to the bathroom pushing the IV pole and readily obliged them, but because I was not told how to prepare it, the nurse told me that I had contaminated the sample with toilet paper. I asked for a bed pan for a second sample and went to the bathroom again and put the smelly sample under a lid outside my cubicle. I now wanted to see the new doctor because the third unit of saline was running out and the Portners would be able to take me home. At this point, the nurse came in, angrily saying that I should not leave the sample out there because it could contaminate others. I had no idea that a bed pan could do this. I apologized, brought the sample back into my cubicle, and asked when I would see the doctor.

"He is doing his rounds now and will see you soon," she said and walked off.

The saline ran out. Susan went off to get the nurse to tell her. She came back and said that they wanted to give me two more units of saline solution more slowly. I said that I wanted to see the doctor before they did this. She asked me if I was refusing treatment. I said that I was not refusing anything but had no idea that they were planning to keep me so long; friends were waiting to take me home. She walked out in a huff. Now that I had been filled with three units of saline solution, I found I had to urinate. I rolled my IV pole out into the corridor, and the nurse said, "Get back to your cubicle! You can't use the bathroom!"

"Why?" I asked

"That's the protocol," she snapped in a nasty, threatening tone.

"What protocol?" I shouted. "No one told me about a protocol. No one told me how to prepare a stool sample. No one told me I was to have a slow IV. And you are being rude to me. Please send the doctor."

A young doctor arrived in my cubicle soon after this outburst.

"How are you feeling?" he said.

"I am perfectly okay. I'm about to go dancing, and I would like to borrow a tuxedo if you have a spare one lying around."

"No need to be sarcastic," he said.

"I've been waiting to see you for over an hour. The IV is finished, and I've submitted my stool sample for analysis, and I think I am about done."

"Your care plan says that you are staying overnight: that's why I thought that there was no hurry to see you. In fact, it says that you were to have two more units of saline solution over the next few hours."

"What care plan?" I said. "No one ever mentioned a care plan to me."

"Also," he continued, "you are on a C-Diff protocol because the doctor thought that you might be infected. There has been an awful lot of it here. Your symptoms are pretty consistent with C. Difficile infection. Even though you are from Toronto, you might have it. That's why you can't go to the bathroom here. I'm really sorry that you weren't told about the care plan or the protocol. He really should have told you before he went home, and there is no excuse for that. So let's do a few more tests to see that you are okay and then we will send you home. I will write you a prescription for a special antibiotic that will deal with the C-Diff if you have it. I will get the results from the stool culture in a day or two. Call me: here is my card with the direct line. Call me on your way back to Toronto. If the test is negative, you can stop taking the antibiotic. I warn you that it is quite expensive."

We got home, and I felt much better. Chaim, my brother-in-law, told me that André Dascal, who is our relative by marriage, had decoded the genetic structure of C. Difficile and was a leading expert on it. We should call him to find out more about the infection. I rested the next day and called André.

André said, "Ooh it sure sounds like C-Diff. You should have called me when you were in the hospital. I would have hurried up the testing. As it is, the lab is now closed for a few days during the holidays, and you'll have to wait for the results. But I have to tell you that there are a lot of false negatives from the short test. I will make sure that your sample is cultured for a week to be sure. I recommend that you take the drug for the full course of treatment."

We went to the drug store to get the antibiotic – it cost $650 for the course of 42 pills. That made it out to a little over $15 a pill. Luckily, it was covered by my private health insurance, but for those not covered, whew.

Eileen Thalenberg, who was in Montreal, agreed to share the driving for our return trip to Toronto. On the way home, we called the hospital for the early results of the test. "It's negative," he said. "You can stop taking the antibiotic."

"Ha!" I thought. Susan won't let me do that now that André has spoken, and I took the full course of the drug.

We got back in time to finish the planning and preparation for our annual New Year's party. I was careful to marshal my energies and took big rests between shopping and preparing for the party. Eileen and Susan did all the setting up. I even went up to rest in bed for several hours during the party.

So my return to life at New Year's was only partial. But I felt like I was returning to normal.

I started swimming again and was regaining the weight that I had lost.

I went back to work on January 2, even though it was still a holiday, because my assistant was returning that day. She needed the money, she said. So I went in and set her to work and stayed for a half day. The theme was that I was half way back.

The next two weeks were uneventful, but the antibiotic made me tired, and my bowel movements (which I now watched carefully) had not returned to normal but remained misshapen, odd-smelling, and somewhat irregular. It's the antibiotic. I also had trouble sleeping. But I went to the gym and swam to get fit again.

Sunday, January 22, 2006: Emergency Room

On the weekend of January 21, I found myself exhausted, and on Sunday, I developed a chest pain that sent me to bed for the afternoon. Rest did not seem to help, so we went once more to the emergency room that night for reassurance: EKG, blood tests, and a chest x-ray – all negative.

Date: 22/01/06
Time: 23:16

EMERGENCY SERVICES (ES) REPORT
DEMOGRAPHICS
Medical Record No.: 2397544
Visit No.: 252054502
Arrival Date: 22/01/2006
Time: 23:16
Brought In By: Family Member
Referred to Physician/Telephone: Joel S. Yaphe/
X3946

ALERT
Presenting Complaint: Chest Pain (CP)
Triage and Acuity Scale: Emergent
Time: 23:12

INVESTIGATIONS
Glucose – 58 mmol/L
Sodium – 141 mmol/L
Potassium – 36 mmol/L
Chloride – 102 mmol/L
Creatinine – 96 mmol/L

DISPOSITION
Discharge Diagnosis: Non-cardiac CP
Attending M.D.: Signature Illegible

HISTORY AND PHYSICAL
Feeling fatigued today. Poor sleep last night. At
noon developed chest pressure. Steady during day
(until now) mild. No cough/Shortness of Breath
(SOB)/None Now.
Laparoscopic Right Hemicolectomy Sept.5, 2005
-      Post-Op Bleed
-      Seen at hospital in Montreal December 5 with
       diarrhea.
-      Rx with Vanco for ? C. Difficile (but) stools
       culture (-)
CRF
-      HTN (mild)
-      Increase in DM, Increase in Cholesterol, no
       Sander
-      Increase 1 degree Pel < 60 with CAD

History (Hx): Cardiovascular Disease
A+O, no distension
Chest Clear
5.5 2 with GR II IV SEN (V) LSB, without illegible
Abdomen soft, no=tender, no L, no S, Bowel
Sounds (BS+)

EKG: Sinus at 57
-      PR = 0.15

ES REPORT CONTINUED

**Date: 22/01/06
Time: 23:16**

- QRC = 0.096
- A 115 (N)
- ST – T(N)

PLAN
Treatment Plan: Labs (N), TN1 negative (-), Chest
X-Ray (CxR) (-)

INTERPRETATION
Impression: Vague chest discomfort, unlikely to be
cardiac:

Discharge (D/C)
Review.

DEM NURSING ASSESMENT

**Date: 22/01/06
Time: 23:12-23:45**

DEPARTMENT OF EMERGENCY MEDICINE
NURSING ASSESSMENT
TGH
Urgent
Date: 22/01/06
Time: 23:12
Present Complaint: Chest Pain (CP)
Triage Assessment: Mid-sternal CP since noon
today. Feeling tired today. CP constant since noon.
Related History: No Shortness of Breath (SOB), no
diaphoresis.
Past Medical History: Colon resection – septic, HTN
Allergies: None Known
Medications: HCTZ, Blood Pressure (BP) medication
Method of Arrival: Ambulatory
Accompanied By: Wife
Triage Nurse Signature: Signature Illegible
Initial Vital Signs
Left Arm Supine: BP 160/75, Pulse (P) 63, Respi-
ratory Rate (RR) 18, Temperature (T) 36, Oxygen
Saturation 98% on RA
Nurse's Signature: Signature Illegible

TimeNurse's Notes
23:30   To x-ray
23:45   Back from x-ray. States had CP since
noon. Mid-sternal. No radiating pain. Felt tired. No
other signs. Denies smoking. Has been tired on and
off for a few weeks. History (Hx) of diarrhea for X 2
days, December 24 and 25. Last bowel movement

DEM ASSESMENT CONTINUED   **Date: 22/01/06
Time: 23:12-23:45**

(BM) today. No peripheral edema. Family history.
Mother died of heart disease. Blood work done by
triage RN well. Family at bedside.
Signature Illegible
Neurological Observation Record/Parameter Record
Date: 22/01/06
Time: 23:45
Coma Scale
Eyes Open = O   (4) Spontaneously
Best Verbal Response = O   (5) Oriented
Best Motor Response = O   (6) Obey Commands
Pupil Scale (m.m.)
Total 15
Blood Pressure and Pulse rate 50-130
Respiration 96% RA

Saturday, January 29, 2006: Infectious Diseases Followup

The continuing fatigue led me to write to Dr. Chan with
what I thought was a question about the C. Difficile.

To: Adrienne Chan
From: Sholom Glouberman
Date: January 29 2006
Subject C Difficile
My name is Seymour (Sholom) Glouberman.
I was your patient at TGH in October of last year as a post
surgical patient who had suffered from "bactericidal."
I tried to get in touch with you after I returned from Montreal
at Christmas. While I was there, I suffered from fainting
and lost control of my bowel and had diarrhea. I went to the
emergency room at the Jewish General Hospital, and after I
give them my history, they put me on a C Difficile protocol.
I was back on antibiotics until January 10. The lab results
were negative, but once more, the infectious diseases doctor at the Jewish General there (Andre Dascal) thought that
it would be a good idea to stay on this course of treatment
anyway.
Since coming off the drugs, I have remained quite tired and
have had occasional bouts of diarrhea.
What do you think are the next steps?
I fear that getting rid of one bug can put me at risk of another.   -Sholom Glouberman

She replied within a couple of days and asked for another stool sample and arranged for yet another CT scan.

> From: Adrienne Chan
> To: Sholom Glouberman
> Date: January 31 2006
> Subject Re C Difficile
> Do you know if there was confirmatory positive C. Difficile toxin? It would be nice to have that result. If you are still having diarrhea then you should come to the hospital and have a C. Difficile test done again. Recurrent C. Difficile can happen when people remain on antibiotics and if they are on immunosuppressant (e.g. steroids). There was an outbreak strain in Quebec (that they have A LOT of experience at the Jewish General with) that seemed to be particularly refractory to treatment. If we document C. Difficile again, you should go on another course of flagyl (metronidazole).
> I am concerned that with the initial negative tests and your ongoing symptoms that something else may be going on. Are you having any fevers, night sweats and abdominal pain? If you aren't busy and you are continuing to have symptoms, I should probably see you (like I can't tell from your story if it is C. diff, or something else, including the abscesses returning). My clinic is usually Friday mornings but if Wednesday mornings are easier I can see you in one of my colleagues' clinics. If you want to come down earlier in the week to get the test done for C. diff then let me know and I will put it in the computer for you to pick up the stool sample in the lab. If you decide to come down this week I will have Deb, our clinic secretary, arrange an appointment for you.
> Best regards,
> Adrienne Chan
> --
> Adrienne K. Chan, MD, FRCPC
> Infectious Diseases Fellow, University of Toronto
> e-mail: adrienne.chan@utoronto.ca
> phone: (416)340-4800 ext 2197 | fax: (416)595-5826

The more sophisticated C. Difficile test turned out to be negative. But now Dr. Chan arranged for one more CT scan on February 14.

The week of February 6, I felt as if I was beginning to get a cold and I stayed home because I was feeling quite unwell. My scalp began to itch, and it became obvious that something was wrong. By Saturday morning, the itch had not gone away and there were also several lumps on my head.

Saturday, February 11, 2006: More Trouble

"Looks like you have some red spots in your scalp," said Susan. "This might be shingles."

I called Telehealth again and the friendly nurse said, "Go see a doctor within the next 24 hours."

We rushed to a walk-in Clinic in our neighbourhood, and shingles it was. I was given an antiviral medication that once more affected my bowel movements but not much else. The itching began to diminish.

Tuesday, February 14, 2006: CT Scan with Shingles

I came to the hospital for my CT scan. The clerk completely ignored me for about ten minutes, and I became quite angry. Then she told me that I should wait in the outside room to get the contrast media that I would have to drink. I was not allowed into the inner area where I had gone before but was led instead to a small room at one side. The clerk in the inner area became rude when I insisted that I be seen at the appointed time and did not respond when I asked why I was put into this small closed room. Incarcerated, I thought, for bad behaviour; I smoldered in this enclosed space. Soon, a friendly technician emerged and apologized for the delay and explained that because I had shingles I had to be kept away from the cancer patients who were vulnerable to infection. I contemplated my good luck and calmed down.

I examined the various pamphlets and found one that requested comments about the scan process. I wrote up the scan that resulted in diarrhea in the ER.

The technician was very friendly and on her best behaviour. She, like the others, warned me of my imminent death at the hands of the CT scanner and then said that I should have some rectally administered contrast fluid. I politely declined.

The results of the CT scan were negative, and Adrienne Chan sent me a full report.

From: Adrienne Chan
To: Sholom Glouberman
Date: February 20 2006
Subject CT Scan Report
Hi,
Your CT report from Tuesday is up in the computer. Essentially, everything looks normal and there is no evidence of anything concerning.
The detailed report states that there is no evidence of recurrent abscess and the anastomosis site between your small and large bowel looks good. There are a large number of diverticula (outpouchings) seen in your large bowel (they apparently were present previously) and there is no evidence of bowel inflammation consistent with active infection like C. difficile (i.e. there is no C. diff). There are cysts (again, benign nothings) in your liver and kidney unchanged from prior scans. It also looks like you have some kidney stones in your left kidney (again unchanged from previously).
Nothing has to be done about the cysts (which are just there), and nothing has to be done about the stones unless you develop renal colic (pain from the stone trying to pass) in the future. Most of the time these stones just stay there and don't cause any trouble but remember that you have them in case you start having left sided flank and/or groin pain in the future, in which case you'd have to have a urologist deal with the stones.
The diverticula in your colon are common and develops as you age and are usually related to weakening and small outpouchings in the colon wall because of chronic constipation. You may actually be constipated without realizing it as it may be the norm for you. Diverticulosis usually isn't problematic, but people with ongoing constipation can develop diverticulitis (inflammation) which presents as crampy abdominal pain and fever +/- diarrhea (so again

something to keep in mind for the future). One wonders if your bout over the holiday may have even been diverticulitis. The best thing to do to prevent the diverticulitis is to have a good bowel routine to keep regularity and soften up your stools. If metamucil is working for you I would recommend that you keep it going as a routine. If you start getting bunged up (ie. not going daily) with the metamucil then add a teaspoon of lactulose (which is a liquid osmotic you can get over the counter...Costco sells them in 1 L bottles).

There is no harm from using metamucil and lactulose chronically (as Dr. Keystone always tells his patients with irritable bowel, he himself has used this regimen for over 20 years!).

Let me know if you have further questions or need to make another appointment.

Best regards,
Adrienne Chan

--
Adrienne K. Chan, MD, FRCPC
Infectious Diseases Fellow, University of Toronto
e-mail: adrienne.chan@utoronto.ca
phone: (416)340-4800 ext 2197 | fax: (416)595-5826

I was finally released from what felt like endless medical supervision. I have since recovered and am back to normal. But the experience has added a new perspective to all my work. I have continued to wonder about the dramatic difference between my experience as a patient and my previous understanding of the world of health care. I still teach and consult in the field. However, the experience of my operation made me see how much the voice of patients needs strengthening and that our perspective must become part of any attempt to improve the health system.

Afterword

March 2006 to December 2009

I began to try to retrieve my medical record in March of 2006 and finally managed to get almost all of it by May with the help of medical friends, helpful nurses, and Sharon Rogers, the patient representative at UHN. Having the record helped me to assemble the memoir and make sure that the dates were accurate. I also discovered some new and interesting details, such as the fact that my appendix was removed. Much of 2006 was spent editing my story, transcribing the record, and trying to make sense of the two. There were many disparities between my experience and what was recorded in the charts. But this was to be expected. The subjective feelings that I had and the objective situation in which my body found itself seemed to be distinct worlds.

In January 2007, I was sent for an echocardiogram. Several days later, my family doctor called and told me that the results showed that there was mild regurgitation in several valves of my heart. This was not a serious condition on its own, but it meant that I would have to take antibiotics before every visit to my dentist to avoid the possibility of infection reaching my heart. I thought no more about this until April when I looked at the manuscript of this memoir, still unsure about what to do with it. I glanced at the results of the echocardiogram during my hospital stay and saw that it too mentioned regurgitation in the valves of my heart. I was no longer complacent. I had already been surprised to find from the record that my appendix had been removed during the operation on my colon. Taking out my appendix without telling me was one thing, but failing to tell me about a condition that put me at risk of serious infection was something that could not be ignored. It was not mere unpleasantness; I had been mistreated and now I would do something about it.

I contacted Sharon Rogers, the patient representative for UHN, and she scheduled a meeting with Richard Reznick, the surgeon who operated on me. Dr. Reznick told me that the valve regurgitation wasn't very serious and that he didn't want to worry me about it at the time. He also assured me that the hospital and he were doing things to improve communication with patients. But given my own experiences, this was little consolation. I called Sharon again to express my concerns, but to my surprise, she told me that the hospital already had procedures in place to do what I suggested. Despite the fact that these procedures were not applied, she was not prepared to think about them or about other ways to improve the patient experience. In the end, it became painfully clear that, fundamentally, her job was to defend the hospital.

Over the next two months, Sharon and I corresponded about these issues at some length, but the results remained the same. Eventually, a meeting was held with Sharon, Dr. Reznick, Bob Bell (the CEO of the hospital), and me. We had a discussion about the hospital's efforts to improve patient satisfaction, and I suggested that the patient perspective really should be part of those efforts. I told them that I had become strongly committed to improving patients' experience in the hospital and would prefer to join them to contribute to their efforts rather fight them from the outside. They agreed, and several months after the meeting, they asked me to join the hospital's Transition Management Team – Patient-Centered Care committee (TMT-PCC). This committee was meant to help the hospital become more focused on patients.

I realized before the first committee meeting that if I was to represent the patient voice then I would need to bring not only my own perspective and experience but that of other patients as well. It was quite easy to find people with personal experience at the receiving end of health care who wanted to help. Everyone was interested, and five friends and colleagues agreed to form a support group to review the meeting with me.

In November 2007, after my first meeting of the TMT-PCC, I collected my impressions and sought the advice of my patient support group. We had a bracing discussion of the nature of the patient experience and the resistance of the system to change. Everyone also had a lot to get off their chest: they all had had one or more difficult encounters with the system and insisted on telling us all about them. Perhaps because of this, we came up with a tentative name for ourselves: "The Group for Realistically Improving Patient Experience" or GRIPE. My sense was that our name was apt. We all felt that there was a lot to gripe about. We all wanted to make things better, and we recognized that this would be no easy task. We knew that the system was resistant to change, yet we were not entirely agreed on what was wrong or what to do about it. These GRIPE discussions were the beginning of a long process that was needed to clarify what we were about, what we wanted to do, and how we wanted to do it. Suggestions included better and easier access to all patient information, better alignment of the various services, and greater involvement of patients in hospital policies regarding clinical care. The discussions were full of emotion, trepidation, and the worry that we might never have much of an impact on the system.

Later that month, I arranged to have a meeting with the hospital's surgical residents to discuss patient-centered care initiatives, and I used the next GRIPE meeting to discuss the best way to approach it. The advice I received was to use the time to explore the residents' own experience of working with patients. The doctors among us were convinced that the experience of being a resident could use improvement. This was a first glimpse of the idea that we might need to work to improve the experience not only of patients but of others involved in health care. Several meetings with residents confirmed this conclusion.

As a member of the TMT-PCC, I was asked to join a web based "Virtual Patient Focus Group," which was occasionally surveyed to elicit patients' perspective on things. I brought the first survey to a GRIPE meeting so that we could respond collectively. By this time, GRIPE membership had begun to grow and included a former Minister of Health and a veteran nurse. We all contributed to the suggestions that were sent back to the survey. The sense that GRIPE might contribute something useful increased. It looked like we were beginning to think together about ways to improve the health care experience.

By the fall, we had begun to articulate how GRIPE should organize itself to be an effective participant in efforts to improve the patient experience, and we began to think of projects to this end. We found, however, that we had vastly different ideas about what to do next. Some felt that a good project might be to increase patient access to their records. Others thought that we should focus on making the availability of care more equitable. Still others thought that we should work towards a new aging-at-home strategy. We were not yet agreed on how to move forward. We did agree that we should find projects that we could all work on. We also saw that we were a good mix of people, and we very much wanted to do something to improve the patient experience. We decided to meet soon after to continue this kind of discussion.

One of the original members of the TMT-PCC support group had had a stroke and needed therapy. He opened the meeting by telling us about a recent good experience he had had with care at the Toronto Rehabilitation Institute, where he was warmly welcomed, seen on time, listened to, carefully treated, and sent on his way. It was an important moment in the development of the group. People who had been brought together through griping were beginning to recognize that there might also be some patient experiences to celebrate, and that our name might be too negative. It was also at this meeting that another early member confessed that she had started a similar organization. She had been waiting to tell us about it because she was not sure that our group was going anywhere. But now we were ready to organize ourselves properly, and she offered us her experience with her very successful startup organization dedicated to non-smokers' rights. She told us that it was important for us to work through our differences and come to a shared agreement about our main objectives and about what we wanted to accomplish.

We have worked hard at many meetings toward this end. The ideas flowed, but at the heart of them were the stories that everyone told about their health care experiences. Everyone we spoke to about our group was sympathetic. Some felt that our objectives were impossible to achieve; others believed that the time had come for a patient led organization to try to improve people's experience with health care. Everyone had illuminating stories to tell.

We recognized that at the core of our efforts must be the collection of patient stories. They express the deeply human interactions that we have experienced in the health care system, the frustrations we have with it, the desire to sympathize with and also flee from other people's pain and suffering. The wide variety of stories and the many twists and unexpected turns that accompany our experiences deepen our understanding of the nature of the patient experience and help us articulate the patient perspective on health care issues.

In the end, it became clear that an association was needed to gather these perspectives, to speak for patients, and to support us in our interactions with the system. We would become a patient led and patient governed organization that brings the patient voice to the health field in order to improve the health care experience for all. We would gather stories and engage in research and educational activities. The Patients' Association of Canada was born.

Recalling now the events surrounding my operation and the subsequent efforts of the Patients' Association, I am reminded of a story that I was told many years ago about a nurse who had worked in a cancer ward. She swore that if she was ever told she had cancer, she would not suffer through the end stages of the disease. She procured a bottle of a powerful pain killer that if drunk at once would be enough to give her a painless death. She carried it with her for many years to remind her of her promise. When she herself was found to have cancer, she was very careful never to ask for a diagnosis, and so was never told that she had the disease. Her death was prolonged and very painful, and the bottle remained untouched at her bedside. Perhaps none of us know how we will behave once we become patients – even when fully armed.

Glossary

Adventitious sounds - Adventitious sounds are never heard over normal lungs but are rather added to normal breath sounds. They can be heard from the lungs themselves or from other parts of the chest, such as pleura or pericardium. They can be discontinuous (crackles) or continuous (wheezes).

Afebrile - The condition of being at optimum temperature (36.8° Celsius); having no fever.

Albumin - The clear fluid portion of the blood. The most abundant plasma protein in humans and other mammals, albumin, is essential for maintaining the osmotic pressure needed for proper distribution of body fluids between intravascular compartments and body tissues.

Allen's Test - Allen's test is a test used to determine the integrity of the blood supply to the hand. With the hand elevated, both the ulnar and the radial arteries are blocked, which leads to blanching (whitening) of the hand. Then, one of the arteries is released, and in the normal case, the blanching disappears over the whole of the hand. This is repeated with both arteries (in theory, the whole of the blood supply of the hand can come from either artery).

Amox - Amoxicillin is used to treat certain infections caused by bacteria, such as pneumonia; bronchitis; gonorrhea; and infections of the ears, nose, throat, urinary tract, and skin. It is also used in combination with other medications to eliminate H. pylori, a bacterium that causes ulcers. Amoxicillin is in a class of medications called penicillin-like antibiotics. It works by stopping the growth of bacteria.

Amox-Clav (Amoxicillin–Clavulanate) - A penicillin antibiotic used to treat a broad-spectrum of bacterial infections, especially resistant strains.

Ampicillin - A beta-lactam antibiotic that has been used extensively to treat bacterial infections since 1961. It can sometimes result in allergic reactions that range in severity from a rash to potentially lethal anaphylaxis.

Amylase - The name given to enzymes that break down starch. They are classified as saccharidases, enzymes that cleave polysaccharides.

Amylase Test - A test to measure the amount of amylase in serum (blood). This test is primarily performed to diagnose or monitor diseases of the pancreas. It may also reflect some gastrointestinal problems.

Anaerobe - Any organism that does not require oxygen for growth. Anaerobes are potentially pathogenic when displaced from normal environments (human colon, soil) and implanted in dead or dying tissue; abscesses, pneumonias, and oral and pelvic infections result.

Anastomosis - A surgical connection between 2 structures. It usually refers to a connection that is created between tubular structures, such as blood vessels or loops of intestine.

Aspirate - To remove liquids or gases by means of a suction device.

Bacteremia - Also known as blood poisoning or toxemia, bacteremia is the presence of bacteria in the blood.

Bacteroides Fragilis - A bacterium that is one of the predominant microorganisms in the lower intestinal tract of humans. The most common member of the normal gut flora, it can cause serious infections if the normal gastrointestinal mucosal barrier is breached. In the bloodstream, the organism can be carried to virtually any organ of the body.

Bilirubin - A breakdown product of hemoglobin. Total and direct bilirubin are usually measured to screen for or to monitor liver or gall bladder dysfunction.

Bolus - A large dose of a medication that is given (usually intravenously by direct infusion injection or gravity drip) at the beginning of treatment to raise blood-level concentrations to a therapeutic level.

Cardiomegaly - A medical condition where the heart is enlarged.

Cardiomyopathy - A weakening of the heart muscle or a change in heart muscle structure. It is often associated with inadequate heart pumping or other heart function abnormalities.

Ceftriaxone - An antibiotic in a class of drugs called cephalosporins. Ceftriaxone fights bacteria in the body. It is used to treat many different types of bacterial infections such as bronchitis, pneumonia, blood infections, bone and joint infections, meningitis, abdominal infections, skin infections, ear infections, gonorrhea, pelvic inflammatory disease, and urinary tract infections.

Coagus - Blood work.

Colace (Docusate Sodium) - Belongs to the family of laxatives known as stool softeners. These medications work by allowing liquids to mix with hard stools. They do not cause bowel movements, but allow for passage of the stool without straining. This is especially important in conditions such as heart disease and any circumstances where passage of stools could be potentially painful.

Computed Topography (CT) Scan - A method of body imaging in which a thin x-ray beam rotates around the patient. Small detectors measure the amount of x-rays that make it through the patient or the particular area of interest.

Cyanosis - The characteristic blue color of the skin observed when the amount of unoxygenated hemoglobin in the blood exceeds 5 grams per 100 millilitres of blood.

Diaphoresis - Excessive sweating commonly associated with shock and other medical emergency conditions.

Dysuria - Painful or difficult urination. Dysuria is most commonly due to bacterial infection of the urinary tract causing inflammation of the bladder (cystitis) or kidney (pyelonephritis).

Ecchymosis - The skin discoloration caused by the escape of blood into the tissues from ruptured blood vessels. Ecchymoses can similarly occur in mucous membranes (for example, in the mouth).

Echocardiogram (Echo) - A test in which ultrasound is used to examine the heart.

Echocardiograph - A non-invasive instrument that employs the differential transmission and reflection of ultrasonic waves to image structural and functional abnormalities of the heart.

Ectopy - An abnormal location or position of an organ or body part.

Electrocardiogram (ECG) - A test that records the electrical activity of the heart. An ECG is used to measure the rate and regularity of heartbeats as well as the size and position of the chambers, the presence of any damage to the heart, and the effects of drugs or devices used to regulate the heart.

Electrocardiograph (EKG or ECG) - Measures the electrical activity of the heartbeat. With each beat, an electrical impulse (or "wave") travels through the heart. This wave causes the muscle to squeeze and pump blood from the heart.

Enterics - Rod-shaped Gram-negative bacteria; most occur normally or pathogenically in intestines.

Epigastric - Of or relating to the anterior walls of the abdomen; lying on or over the stomach.

Expectorate - The ejection of saliva, mucous, or other body fluids from the mouth; to clear out the chest and lungs by coughing up and spitting out matter.

Fentanyl - Belongs to the group of medicines called narcotic analgesics, which are used to relieve pain.

Flagyl (Metronidazole) - An antibiotic used to treat abdominal infections.

Foley Catheter - A self-retaining tube placed through the urethra into the bladder for continuous urine drainage.

Genitourinary - Concerning the organ system of all the reproductive organs and the urinary system.

Glasgow Coma Scale - A scale for measuring the level of consciousness in which scoring is determined by three factors: amount of eye opening, verbal responsiveness, and motor responsiveness.

Gram-Negative Bacteria - Bacteria that do not retain crystal violet dye in the Gram staining protocol. Gram-positive bacteria will retain the dark blue dye after an alcohol wash, whereas Gram-negative do not. In a Gram stain test, a counter-stain is added after the crystal violet, which colors all Gram-negative bacteria a red or pink color. The test itself is useful in classifying two distinctly different types of bacteria based on structural differences in their cell walls.

Haemotology - The science encompassing the medical study of the blood and blood-producing organs. Haem is a complex red organic pigment containing iron and other atoms to which oxygen binds.

Hematoma - A collection of blood, generally the result of hemorrhage, or, more specifically, internal bleeding. Hematomas exist as bruises (ecchymoses), but can also develop in organs.

Hematuria - The presence of red blood cells (RBCs) in the urine. In microscopic hematuria, the urine appears normal to the naked eye, but examination under a microscope shows a high number of RBCs. Gross hematuria can be seen with the naked eye – the urine is red or the color of cola.

Hemicolectomy - A procedure where a portion of the left or right large bowel is removed due to the presence of cancer. This is done through a large incision in the abdominal wall. The affected area of the bowel is removed and the two remaining ends joined together.

Hemodynamics - The study of the properties and flow of blood.

Hemoptysis - Spitting up blood or blood-tinged sputum.

Heparin - An anticoagulant used to decrease the clotting ability of the blood and help prevent harmful clots from forming in the blood vessels.

Homan's Sign - An indicator of deep venous thrombosis. The sign is present where pain in the calf is produced by passive dorsiflexion of the foot.

Ileus - Intestinal obstruction involving a partial or complete blockage of the bowel that results in the failure of the intestinal contents to pass through.

Incentive Spirometer - Used to examine the health of lungs by measuring inspiratory volume. Specifically, measures how well lungs are filled with each breath.

Interventional Radiology - A subspecialty of radiology in which minimally invasive procedures are performed using image guidance. Some of these procedures are done for purely diagnostic purposes, while others are done for treatment purposes. Pictures are used to direct these procedures, which are usually done with needles or other tiny instruments such as catheters. The images allow Interventional Radiologists to guide these instruments through the body to the areas of interest.

Intraperitoneal - Within the peritoneal cavity, the area that contains the abdominal organs.

Irrigate - To supply with a constant flow or sprinkling of liquid for the purpose of cooling, cleansing, or disinfecting,

Keflex - An antibiotic in a class of drugs called cephalosporins. Keflex fights bacteria in the body and is used to treat many different types of bacterial infections such as bronchitis, tonsillitis, ear infections, skin infections, and urinary tract infections.

Lactated Ringer's Solution - An intravenous (IV) solution used to supply water and electrolytes (e.g., calcium, potassium, sodium, chloride), either with or without calories (dextrose). It is also used as a mixing solution (diluent) for other IV medications.

Laparoscopic - Refers to operations within the abdomen or pelvic cavity.

Lasix (Furosemide) - Furosemide belongs to the class of medications called diuretics. Diuretics like furosemide are used for the treatment of edema (fluid retention) that occurs with congestive heart failure and disorders of the liver, kidney, and lungs. It is also used to control high blood pressure. Furosemide increases the amount of urine produced and excreted and removes excessive water (edema).

Left Ventricular Hypertrophy - The abnormal thickening of the myocardium (muscle) of the left ventricle of the heart.

Maxiflor - A brand name for Diflorasone, a topical steroid. Maxiflor reduces or inhibits the actions of chemicals in the body that cause inflammation, redness, and swelling.

Melena - Refers to the black, "tarry" feces that are associated with gastrointestinal hemorrhage. The black color is caused by oxidation of the iron in hemoglobin during its passage through the ileum and colon.

Moxiflox - Moxifloxacin is a synthetic fluoroquinolone antibiotic agent.

Nocturia - Being awoken at night by the excessive need for urination.

Ostomy - An operation to create an opening from an area inside the body to the outside.

Peritonitis - Peritonitis is an inflammation (irritation) of the peritoneum, the tissue that lines the wall of the abdomen and covers the abdominal organs.

Premature Ventricular Contraction - An extra heartbeat resulting from abnormal electrical activation originating in the ventricles before a normal heartbeat would occur.

Pruritus - An itching feeling.

Rigor - Shaking occurring during a high fever.

Sanguineous - Containing, secreting, or resembling blood.

Seropurulent - Consisting of a mixture of serum and pus.

Serous Sanguineous (Sero-sang/Serous-sang) - Consisting of serum and blood.

Serous - Containing, secreting, or resembling serum.

Sputum - A secretion that is produced in the lungs and the bronchi (tubes that carry the air to the lung). This mucus-like secretion may become infected, bloodstained, or contain abnormal cells that may lead to a diagnosis. Sputum is often produced by deep coughing.

Steri-strips - Strips of tape that are placed across an incision to keep the edges of the wound together as it heals.

Sublingual - Under the tongue.

Supine - Lying face upwards.

Syncope/Syncopal Episodes - A transient loss of consciousness with an inability to maintain postural tone that is followed by spontaneous recovery. The term syncope excludes seizures, coma, shock, or other states of altered consciousness.

Telemetry - The science and technology of automatic measurement and transmission of data by wire, radio, or other means from remote sources to receiving stations for recording and analysis.

The Stress Echo Test - Combines an echocardiogram (cardiac ultrasound) with a stress test to assess the performance of the heart at rest and under stress. This information helps to determine if there are any blockages or narrowings in the coronary arteries (coronary artery disease), which supply blood to heart muscles. Coronary artery disease may lead in turn to chest pain (angina) and heart attack.

Tonsillectomy and Adenoidectomy - The surgical removal of the tonsils and adenoids.

Toradol (Ketorolac oral) - Ketorolac belongs to the class of medications called nonsteroidal anti-inflammatory drugs (NSAIDs). It is used for the short-term treatment of moderate to moderately severe acute pain after surgery and works by reducing pain, swelling, and inflammation.

Trendelenburg Position - Position in which the patient is on an elevated and inclined plane, usually about 45°, with the head down and legs and feet over the edge of the table. It is used in abdominal operations to push abdominal organs towards the chest.

Troponin Tests - Primarily performed on patients who have chest pain to determine occurence of heart attack or other damage to the heart.

Urometer - An instrument used to measure urine concentration.

Vasovagal Reaction - A reflex of the involuntary nervous system that causes the heart to slow down. A vasovagal reaction also affects the nerves to the blood vessels in the legs, thereby permitting those vessels to dilate (widen). As a result, the heart pumps less blood, blood pressure drops, and what blood is circulating tends to go into the legs rather than to the head. The brain is deprived of oxygen and a fainting episode usually results. The vasovagal reaction is also called a vasovagal attack. The resultant fainting is synonymous with situational syncope, vasovagal syncope, and vasodepressor syncope.

Versed (Midazolam) - Used to produce sleepiness or drowsiness and to relieve anxiety before surgery or certain procedures. It is also used to produce loss of consciousness before and during surgery. Midazolam is sometimes used for patients in intensive care units in hospitals to cause unconsciousness. This may allow the patients to withstand the stress of being in the intensive care unit and help the patients cooperate when a machine must be used to assist them with breathing.

Villous Adenoma - A usually solitary, large, often sessile tumor of the mucosa of the large intestine composed of mucinous epithelium covering delicate vascular projections.

Zantac - A class of drugs called histamine receptor antagonists. Zantac works by decreasing the amount of acid the stomach produces. It is used to treat and prevent ulcers in the stomach and intestines, as well as to treat conditions in which the stomach produces too much acid and conditions in which acid rises to the esophagus and causes heartburn.

CPSIA information can be obtained at www.ICGtesting.com
232764LV00004B/105/P

9 780981 261805